CANCER HEALED NATURALLY

MY JOURNEY FROM BREAST CANCER TO VIBRANT HEALTH

DANIELLE WOTHERSPOON

Copyright © 2018 by Danielle Wotherspoon

All rights reserved. No part of this book may be reproduced, stored in retrieval systems or transmitted by any means, electronic, mechanical, photocopying recorded or otherwise without written permission from the author.

**How to order this book: Amazon.com.
also available at
www.naturalhealthjourneys.org**

Dedication

To my husband Bruce and my son Jonathan who supported my journey even though you thought some of my healing methods were rather unconventional at times.

Praise for Cancer Healed Naturally

Dr. Herman Spies - 15 June 2018.

If we consider that symptoms and disease are our body's way of telling us that something that we do or think is harming us, then it follows that to improve the situation, we have to start doing things differently.

For many years, patients have handed the management of their health to a "more qualified and knowledgeable" person. This approach left the patient disempowered, trusting somebody else to fix their problem for them. Therefore, their own ability to change the situation was ignored/undermined.

My job as a medical practitioner is to teach all my patients that their health is in their own hands. You may outsource some aspects of your treatment to someone with more knowledge/experience for a certain purpose or period of time, but the patient should always be in control of their healing journey. They have to learn the lessons and/or make the necessary changes to their lifestyle, habits, thinking or diet.

It is therefore so refreshing to meet a patient like Danielle, because she immediately understood that she was responsible for her healing journey. It is clear from her journey that she took ownership of her own health, and how she was prepared to make the necessary changes to allow her body to heal again.

Her determination to get to the bottom of what her disease was trying to tell her, put her on a path of self growth that enriched the lives of her family and herself in a multitude of ways.

I am sure that each reader will be as inspired and empowered by her journey as I was when I read it.

Dr. Herman Spies,
M.B.Ch.B., M.B.A., DFHon, Dip. Acup,
Homotox.
26 Olienhout Avenue, Plattekloof, Cape Town,
Tel: (021) 930 6023 | **Mobile**: (082) 577 6320
Website: www.drspies.com | **Email**: doc@drspies.com

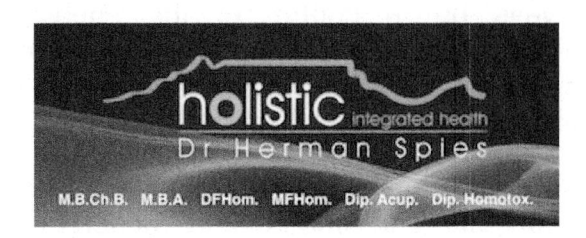

Suret Morkel - 6 May 2018

I am so impressed by your book! It is lovely to read about the many healing modalities you pursued.

This book is going to be of great value not only to every person who wants to know more, but also to many a practitioner who needs to know more about "healing the natural way"

I so enjoyed reading your book, and especially the following aspects:
- Your recipes – such as The Turmeric drinks.
- Lymph self-massages - a beautiful recommendation - with no added expenses!
- The trampoline rebounder for exercise and relaxation.
- The castor oil packs for revitalising the liver and daily intake of iodine - so important for natural thyroid hormone production.
- Coffee enemas and colonic irrigations which I also believe are integral parts of a natural anti-cancer treatment plan.
- The way you compartmentalized the book with rather short and easily readable chapters describing what you did and included an extended list of references for those who want to know where you gained all this lovely knowledge - which compounded into fabulous reading material.
- Your section on the love of God for us
- And laughter - a healing modality!

- The section on prayer – as I know that our healthy bodies vibrate at 68 MHz per second, but, when we pray, our vibration frequency raises by 13 MHz.

Suret Morkel,
Medical Scientist, Microbiologist
Natural health practice number: 7591713

Physical Address: 9 Skoonlief street, Kuils River,
Tel: 0861779977 **Mobile:** 073 9000 347
Website: www.innerfruits.com **Email:** suret@innerfruits.com

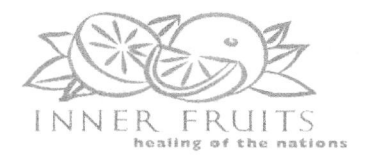

INNER FRUITS
healing of the nations

Table of Contents

Dedication ii

Praise for Cancer Healed Naturally iii

Table of Contents vii

Disclaimer xi

1. Introduction 1

2. An Unexpected Discovery and a
   Frightening Diagnosis 5

3. Why Cancer in My Body? 12

   A. General Risk Factors 12

   B. Other Risk Factors 14

4. Reasons for not selecting Radiation
   or Chemotherapy 21

   A. Survival Rate 22

   B. Side Effects 26

   C. Cancer Stem Cells Survive Radiation
      and Chemotherapy 29

5. High-Dose Intravenous Vitamin C–My Primary Treatment. 32

6. Treatment Protocols by an Integrated Health Professional 40

   A. High-Dose Intravenous Vitamin C Drips 41

   B. Electromagnetic Homeopathic Solutions..42

   C. Supplements and Herbs 43

   D. Footbaths 46

   E. Rife Resonator Machine 47

   F. Other Protocols recommended by Dr Spies 47

7. My Cancer-Fighting Diet..49

   A. Why I Chose a Vegan Diet 50

   B. Cancer -Fighting Foods 55

   C. Juicing and Digestion 67

   D. Further Steps to Improve Digestion and Get the Nutrients You Need 71

   E. Organic Fruits and Vegetables.....................................73

F. ORAC (Oxygen Radical Absorbance Capacity)..75

G. My Typical Daily Vegan Menu...................77

H. Evolving My Anti-Cancer Maintenance Diet 82

8. The Gut and Cancer..96

   A. Cancer Gut Bacteria Connection....................97

   B. Foods to Restore the Gut. 99

9. Parasites and Cancer 103

10. Coffee Enemas for Detoxification 108

   A. History of the Coffee Enema 108

   B. Making and Using a Coffee Enema 110

11. Lymphatic System and Drainage Methods 113

   A. Gentle Lymph Self-Massage 116

   B. Lymph Pressure Massage or Air Therapy..118

   C. Rebounding on a Small Trampoline 119

   D. Water 120

- E. Castor Oil Packs 121
- F. Infrared and Ozone Saunas 122
- G. Exercise 124
12. Thyroid and Iodine Connection 128
    - A. The Functions of Iodine in the Body. 130
    - B. Iodine Deficiency and Breast Cancer 131
13. Emotions and Stress 134
14. The Importance of My Faith in God 145
    - A. Discovering the Father's Love 146
    - B. The story of King Hezekiah 148
    - C. My Dream 150
    - D. Spiritual Disciplines that Helped me on my Healing Journey 151
15. Conclusion 164

Acknowledgements. 168

Addendum A 172

References 175

Disclaimer

This book is not to be construed as giving any specific medical advice. It reflects the choices I made in consultation with an integrative medical practitioner – Dr Spies, who treated me for a period, and gave me certain of the protocols outlined in the book.

The remainder of the choices and protocols I followed were based on my own research I undertook and feedback from Dr Spies and others.

Each case is different and requires that you need to assess what is available and consult a medical practitioner. Should you decide to go the journey I went on, you will require a qualified integrative medical practitioner to give you guidance.

1. Introduction

Receiving the diagnosis of cancer is a shattering experience. To add to this, in my case, the doctor making the diagnosis made it clear that if I did not heed the instructions to use surgery, chemotherapy and/or radiation, I would more than likely die. The conventional oncology industry wants a person diagnosed with cancer to commit as soon as possible to entering into the conventional treatment protocols.

The purpose of this book is to share my journey of overcoming breast cancer through the use of natural and alternative methods, in lieu of those predominantly used today. Most methods involve the use of chemotherapy and radiation, either individually or in combination. I will be sharing in detail everything I did to restore my health since the diagnosis of infiltrating ductal carcinoma of the left breast, and metastatic ductal carcinoma in the left lymph node.

During this process I have not only added ten good, healthy years to my life, but I also have more energy now at 61 than when I was 45. In addition, the eczema that plagued me since childhood has cleared up.

The truth is that a cancer diagnosis is not generally a medical emergency. You have time to consider your options and decide which treatment is best suited to you. The diagnosis of cancer need not be seen as a death sentence or an automatic prescription for chemotherapy and radiation. I want to show you, through the healing journey described in this book, that you can take charge of your own life and health.

There are a number of alternative therapies that can be used successfully. Many have been scientifically proven to assist in natural, gentle and more affordable ways to heal cancer, while avoiding the debilitating side effects of chemotherapy and radiation. The conventional treatments kill more than just the cancer cells; weaken the immune system and increase inflammation in the body. Therefore, cancer patients can take up to two years or more to recover after the chemotherapy treatment before they feel well again.

During my treatment period I never suffered from side effects that hindered me from undertaking my basic, everyday activities. I was able to continue with my life as normal. In fact, I was doing so well that I could travel overseas to Europe after seven months after commencing my treatment.

I didn't tell many people about the breast cancer diagnosis. The main reason for not sharing this was the overarching societal view that "cancer untreated with conventional means leads to death". I didn't want this mantra to be spoken over me.

In addition, many would have tried to convince me to follow the chemotherapy route. I know of a number of people who started out on the natural route, but were persuaded by pressure from loved ones, friends and doctors to change to conventional treatment. Most of my close family and friends, whom I told of my choice, to this day still don't understand what my journey entailed - which was another reason for sharing my experiences in this book.

Cancer develops in a person's body because of a compromised immune system. The protocols I used were all focused on repairing and recharging the immune system to an optimal level. Only then was my body equipped to heal cancer naturally.

Even if you decide to undergo chemotherapy and radiation, the alternative therapies that I used can work in conjunction with these, to assist your immune system and therefore speed up your recovery. The moral of the story: there are alternatives out there that can work as effectively as chemotherapy and radiation. You can allow your diagnosis to de-capacitate you, or propel you forward into becoming a more healthy and whole person. Besides the wonderful health benefits I gained from my journey, I also grew in wisdom, faith and character.

Remember that a cancer diagnosis is NOT a death sentence.

It can, however, be the beginning of one of the most transformative periods of your life. It has definitely been life-changing for me. I can truthfully say that I'm mentally and emotionally healthier.

The first-hand experience I gained on my healing journey compelled me to share my discoveries in this book, which I have named *Cancer Healed Naturally*, for reasons which will become clearer and more understandable as you read further.

2. An Unexpected Discovery and a Frightening Diagnosis

It was late afternoon January 2, 2008. We had just returned from our annual holiday on the Garden Route, near George. It had been very challenging, owing to my husband, Bruce's, struggles with his health at the time. He'd suddenly become very ill in late November the previous year, and we were still unsure about the cause for this sudden onset of ill-health.

He was suffering from many incapacitating symptoms, like severe dizzy spells and an inability to concentrate. His heart rate dropped from its normal rate of 60 to 35; he also suffered from inflamed mucous membranes, which caused a permanently sore throat. His immune system became compromised and he had very low energy. He turned from a healthy, active man that could surf and participate in various other sports, to someone who couldn't walk on the beach unassisted, because of the dizzy spells and abnormally low heart rate.

This all started after a dentist removed nine of the amalgam fillings from his teeth, in one sitting, without taking any precautions. The doctors and specialists that he saw (and there were a number of them) couldn't figure out what was wrong. Even though we mentioned the amalgam filling episode, they chose to ignore it. They were looking for conventional reasons.

A friend of ours, Colleen, suggested that a misalignment of his jaw might be causing the dizzy spells, and recommended that he see a holistic dentist, Dr Pieter Cilliers, from De Necker Dentistry.

Dr Cilliers immediately recognised Bruce's symptoms as mercury poisoning, especially against the background of the removal of the nine amalgam fillings. He recommended Dr Herman Spies in Cape Town, an integrative holistic medical doctor. Dr Spies was to become instrumental in leading Bruce (and later on, myself) back to health.

So, there I was, enjoying a shower after the long, six-hour journey home. I had to drive most of the way, because of Bruce's condition. It felt great to be showering off all the grime and stress after the journey. I was looking forward to a good night's sleep.

While applying some cream to my body I felt a sizable lump on the side of my left breast. Fear gripped my heart, and, in my mind, I cried out, "It surely can't be? How did I miss the lump in the past?"

I remembered looking at a special insurance policy for breast cancer that'd received via post a while before. It would cover all the additional expenses in the case of someone being diagnosed with cancer, like extra hospital costs, a personal caregiver and even a convalescent home if you needed one after your chemotherapy. I'd thrown it in the bin then because I'd thought to myself, "I am definitely not a candidate for breast cancer." (The thought "what if?" did surface for a moment, however.)

So I held on to a sense of comfort that it could not be malignant, taken from the perception I had that didn't fit the typical cancer profile – my reasoning went something along the lines that:
- I wasn't overweight and was actually more on the lean side.
- I didn't smoke.
- I didn't use alcohol, except for a glass of wine on a special occasion.
- I was exercising daily.
- I was eating lots of mostly organic, fresh fruit, vegetables and legumes.
- I consumed very few animal products.
- I followed a diet that was sugar and wheat-free.
- I made vegetable juice almost daily.
- I was using some supplements as well.

So, I thought I was really living a healthy lifestyle. I had discovered in my thirties that it was the best thing to do to control the eczema I had suffered from since birth.

I was, however, easily stressed and tired quickly.

I decided initially not to go for any tests. Firstly, because I felt that I couldn't share my discovery with my husband as he was too fragile health-wise and I couldn't risk loading him with an additional burden. Second, I wasn't feeling sick or experiencing any pain and was comfortably functional. So I didn't tell anyone about the lump for about six months.

My time was taken up by the household, assisting Bruce with his healing and taking care of our son Jonathan, who was 15 years old at the time. I suppressed my fear of the lump being cancerous. It should not be malignant, I kept trying to reassure myself, but a slight sense of doubt and caution cropped up on occasion.

Eventually I decided to consult a friend of mine, Suret Morkel. Suret is a biomedical scientist, microbiologist and natural healthcare practitioner, and has been working in the areas of diet, detoxification, fresh raw food, fresh juice fasting, supplements and high-dose vitamin C intravenous drips since 1996

She initially recommended that I have eight grams of specially compounded 500mg/ml vitamin C injected once a week, directly into the veins of the arms. We hoped that the antioxidant properties of vitamin C would assist in reducing the size of the lump, and hopefully lead to its complete disappearance.

Suret also recommended that I go for prayer at Healing Rooms. Healing Rooms were initially started in Spokane Washington in 1919, by John G. Lake, to pray for sick people. Many documented healings took place at these rooms. Interestingly, a venue for Healing Rooms had opened in my area a few months before, and I had been there for prayer for the eczema that was playing up at that stage because of stress.

I saw the existence of Healing Rooms so close by, as God's provision. I am a committed Christian, and besides using the vitamin C, was trusting God to heal the lump completely.

But the lump didn't disappear or, for that matter, get any smaller. In actual fact it felt bigger to the touch. Looking back now, I understand that if you want vitamin C to be effective against cancer, you have to follow the correct protocol for high-dose intravenous vitamin C (outlined in this book in chapter 5).

October that year I went to a breast health centre to have a core needle biopsy and ultrasound taken, without a mammogram. I believe that mammograms are not good for you (Mayo Clinic, 2008)[1]. The test results came back inconclusive. The definite nature of the cells tested could not be identified as cancerous or benign.

The doctor recommended that I come back for a mammogram, and that I have an excision biopsy, to be sent to the lab for further testing. This involved conscious sedation and a day in theatre. I couldn't do it at that stage as I still hadn't told Bruce. about the lump in my breast.

Bruce, however, was on the mend with the treatment he'd received from Dr Herman Spies. At the beginning of December 2008, 11 months later, I decided I could share my issue with him. It was a huge shock to him, and after much deliberation, prayer and consultation we decided to do the mammogram and excision biopsy. We wanted to at least know what the diagnosis was.

I went back to the breast health centre on January 8, 2009, almost a full year after initially discovering the lump in my breast. I had the ultrasound and mammogram done. I was shocked by the outcome. Not only had the lump in the breast grown from 1.5 cm to 1.9 cm, but there was also a lump in the lymph node under the arm, 2 cm in size.

The excision biopsy took place on January 23, 2009. The biopsy went smoothly, and I recovered very quickly with minimal pain, but waiting to hear the results from the lab tests was unnerving.

The clinic phoned me to make an appointment to see the surgeon, and I was immediately concerned when they wouldn't tell me over the phone what the results were. The results from the tests confirmed that I had a grade one infiltrating (invasive) ductal carcinoma of the left breast and a metastatic ductal carcinoma in the left lymph node of the armpit. The surgeon immediately wanted to schedule a wide local excision (WLE) and an auxiliary lymph node dissection. This was to be followed by radiotherapy and chemotherapy, and possibly hormonal and biological therapy.

At that moment it felt like a death.sentence had been spoken over me. I wanted to burst out crying, and though I was struggling hard to keep my composure, I asked her about the pros and cons of the conventional treatment. I drove away from there, stopping the car a few times because I was crying so bitterly. I felt shattered and shocked by the outcome.

I just couldn't believe that this was happening to me.

3. Why Cancer in My Body?

The nagging question that most people have after being diagnosed with cancer is "Why me?" I earnestly started to search for factors that could have contributed to the manifestation of cancer in my body. The medical profession tells you that it is mostly genetic, so the answers to my questions weren't immediately obvious to me.

The complexity of the answers became more apparent as I completed the many natural protocols I adopted to heal the cancer. I found that the answers to the pertinent question of 'why me' included gaining.an understanding of the emotions I felt and my spiritual state.

A. General Risk Factors

Here is a summary of the risk factors for breast cancer, identified by the University of San Francisco[1]:
- Other breast disease
- Previous breast irradiation
- Abnormal menstrual periods (If you started menstruating before age 12 or if you went through menopause after age 50, your risk is slightly increased.)
- Not having children or if you had your first child after age 30, your risk for breast cancer is slightly increased.

- or if you've not had children or had your first child after age 30, your risk for breast cancer is slightly increased.)
- Not breastfeeding (Your breast cancer risk may be slightly lowered if you breastfeed.)
- Hormone replacement therapy (Long-term use of ten years or more may slightly increase the risk of breast cancer.)
- Alcohol (This is clearly linked to an increased risk for breast cancer. Those who have two to five alcoholic drinks daily have 1.5 times the risk of developing breast cancer as women who do not drink.)
- Weight and diet (Women who are overweight, especially after menopause, are at increased risk for breast cancer. Researchers believe that this is because fat tissue can make oestrogen, and exposure to oestrogen is linked to breast cancer.)
- Physical activity (Recent studies indicate that even moderate exercise may help to lower your breast cancer risk.)
- Exposure to environmental pollutants
- Family history (If you have a close blood relative: a mother or sister who has had breast cancer, your own risk of developing the disease doubles.)
- Age (About 77 percent of women are over age 50 at the time they are diagnosed with breast cancer; less than one percent are diagnosed in their twenties.)

- Oral contraceptives (A recent analysis showed that women who took oral contraceptives in the long term - for more than 12 years-had a slightly higher risk of breast cancer than women who did not take oral contraceptives. Once women stopped taking oral contraceptives for 10 years, their risk appeared to return to the baseline, average risk.)

Based on the above, the following factors could have contributed to my breast cancer:
- Having my first child at 36.
- Being over age 50 (I was 51 years old when diagnosed.)
- Using contraceptives for more than two years.

B. Other Risk Factors
I. Diet
A recent study (Harris, Willet, Vaidya & Michels, (2017)[2] states:

> In conclusion, we observed an association between an adolescent and early adulthood inflammatory dietary pattern, characterized by high intake of sweetened and diet soft drinks, refined grains, red and processed meat, margarine, corn, and fish, and lower intake of green leafy vegetables, cruciferous vegetables, and coffee and the risk of premenopausal breast cancer.

It is clear that a diet that consists of highly inflammatory foods could contribute to breast cancer later on in our lives.

My diet during my twenties and early thirties was highly inflammatory, and the effects of this were now being felt. During my single years, I hardly ever prepared fresh meals at home. I lived on canteen and restaurant food. The only items of food to be found in my fridge were yogurt, bread, margarine, cheese and possibly some apples. Because of this high carbohydrate diet, I also became anaemic at times and needed to take iron supplements.

This could have been another reason for the breast cancer.

II. Iron Imbalance

Xi Huang PhD (2008)[3] came to the following conclusion:

> Iron imbalance is a unique physiological occurrence in women, which is likely to affect health before, during, and after menopause. The possibility exists that iron deficiency contributes to the high recurrence of breast cancer in premenopausal women, whereas iron load might have a role in the incidence of breast cancer in postmenopausal women. Understanding the role of iron imbalance in breast cancer could lead to adjuvant therapeutic treatments, and potentially benefit

patients by decreasing recurrence and incidence and increasing overall survival.

III. The Iodine Factor

I also discovered another reason for the breast cancer in book by Dr David Brownstein MD (2014).[4] The book is about the importance of iodine in female hormones and reproductive organs. He stresses the dangers of taking thyroid medication without adding iodine to the diet. This is an overlooked factor by most medical professionals, as well as by many integrative and alternative medical practitioners.

I had started to use thyroid medication two years before the diagnosis. Based on Dr David Brownstein's studies, regular intake of iodine then became one of my protocols. (For detailed information on this see the section on the thyroid and iodine in chapter thirteen, titled *Thyroid and Iodine Connection*.)

IV. Bilharzia Parasite

According to Jens Rupp,[5] bilharzia is a disease, in humans, caused by parasitic worms called schistosomes:

> Over one billion humans are at risk worldwide, and approximately 300 million are infected. Parasite larvae enter through the skin; the human then becomes their definitive host in whom they mature and reproduce. The worms feed on red blood cells and dissolved nutrients,

such as sugars and amino acids. This can cause anaemia, extreme tiredness and decreased resistance to other diseases.

I had been diagnosed as anaemic since my early twenties, and during my forties suffered from extreme tiredness, but had never been tested for bilharzia. Doctor Herman Spies identified the presence of this parasite in my body through the QUANTEC® scan. Dr Spies (2018)[6] states the following:

> The QUANTEC® uses an original digital photograph of the patient to scan the human body's energy field to identify any existing disorders on an electro-magnetic level. The QUANTEC® scans more than 50 000 remedies in over 200 databases for a response. All three levels - physical, mental and spiritual are assessed. Databases available are for example: colours, sounds, acupuncture, affirmations, allergens, ICD 10 codes, homeopathic remedies, nosodes, Bach flowers, psycho-kinesiology, tissue salts, enzymes, etc.

He told me at our first appointment that he believed that the bilharzia parasite was one of the main causes of my breast cancer.

V. Emotions

Dr Jimenez works with cancer patients all the time. In a conversation with Ty Bollinger (author of *The*

Truth about Cancer), he speaks about detoxification for cancer and says the following:[7]

> A negative thought can kill you faster *than* a bad germ. One of the main things to detoxify is the mind - the emotions, the conflicts and the traumas going back. Detoxifying those psychological, emotional, biological conflicts, and trauma, is key. Then we can talk about other things to detoxify. One of the most important ways you can contribute to your healing is through your own emotional healing.

My health took a quantum leap after I started to work on the negative beliefs that affected my emotions and stress levels. I now believe that emotions that kept me in permanent state of fight-or-flight mode, and therefore in a state of stress, were a major factor contributing to the breast cancer

This topic is discussed in detail under the following titles in chapter twelve: *Emotions* and *Stress*.

VI.   Stress

Heid (2014)[8] quotes a number of doctors in his article on stress and cancer. Here is an excerpt:

> But long-term or chronic stress is more damaging. That type of stress springs from situations that last many weeks or months with no definite end point. "Caring for a sick loved one or dealing with a long stint of unemployment are common causes of chronic stress," Cohen says.

This type of no-end-in-sight stress can weaken your immune system, leaving you prone to diseases like cancer. It also ups your risk for digestive problems and depression. "Chronic stress also can help cancer grow and spread in a number of ways," Sood says: Stress hormones can inhibit a process called anoikis, which kills diseased cells and prevents them from spreading, Sood says.

Chronic stress also increases the production of certain growth factors that increase your blood supply. This can speed up the development of cancerous tumors, he adds.

In my case, for fourteen years I worked as a buyer for a large retail chain. This involved a lot of local and international travel, putting together of clothing ranges for the upcoming seasons, presentations and then negotiations to fix the prices for the manufacture of the goods.

These negotiations involved large amounts of money. Once I left the business, there still seemed to be an underlying tension in my life and I was easily stressed by the smallest incident.

The sudden onset of ill-health in my husband Bruce brought another element of stress into my life. He was a practicing architect with a business he had started a few years earlier.

The business was very dependent on his input to continue functioning as a profitable entity, from which our family could draw an income.

I also did not understand at the time, that much of this stress I was experiencing was due to emotional issues I had experienced in the past and never taken the time to gain understanding of it.

4. Reasons for not selecting Radiation or Chemotherapy

Before deciding on a treatment for my cancer I did as much research as possible, and will elaborate on some of it in this chapter. I will discuss the survival rate of patients after doing chemo, possible side effects from the chemotherapy itself and finally that it is possible for the cancer to re-emerge after completing the chemotherapy itself.

Based on this research and some deep thought and consideration, I decided to not to undergo chemotherapy or radiation treatment.

The surgeon was rather shocked to hear this and asked me to reconsider my choice. She explained that in her view. if I didn't do the radiation and chemotherapy, the possibility that I would die within five years would be high.

But when I asked her about the life span after chemotherapy and radiation, she said she could only guarantee me five years anyway.

It is well known that chemotherapy and radiation severely affect the body and immune system. It can take years to completely detoxify the body of all the poisons given through these conventional treatments.

Furthermore, to predict with certainty when death will occur, if conventional treatment is not followed, is not actually factually correct.

Doctors need to be aware of the manner in which they make pronouncements after diagnosis. The words spoken over a cancer patient can greatly contribute to a sense of insecurity and affect the emotional condition of the patient even further.

My deep love for my wonderful son, and only child, Jonathan, was a huge motivator for me to get healed. I wanted to tackle this challenge with everything I could muster. He was only 15 years old at the time and I wanted to be there for him, as a mother, until he reached full maturity and independence.

So, to do that I had to be fully functional. I also didn't want him to experience the pain of losing a mother at such a young age.

A. Survival Rate

As stated earlier my goal was to combat the cancer, and after having conquered it, to be healthier and stronger than before I was even diagnosed. Therefore the first studies I looked at were the survival rate for patients who undertook chemotherapy. The studies use a term known as the 'five year survival rate' which is quite simply the percentage of people who survive for five years after having undergone chemotherapy.

At the time of my diagnoses, the studies that I found on the five year survival rate painted a very bleak picture for actually doing the chemotherapy. These studies were completed by Morgan, Ward and Barton (2004) and Gawler (2007) and some of the results will be summarized below.

Morgan, Ward and Barton (2004)[2] did an analysis of the five year survival rate after chemotherapy of 22 types of cancer (including breast cancer) in Australia. What shocked me tremendously at the time, was that this study concluded that the five year survival rate for those studied was a low 2.3 percent. They state:

> The minimal impact on survival in the more common cancers conflicts with the perceptions of many people who feel they are receiving a treatment that will significantly enhance their chances of cure. While newer chemotherapy regimes (including taxanes and anthracyclines) may increase survival by one percent at the expense of the risk of cardiac toxicity and nerve damage, to date there is no convincing evidence that newer and more expensive regimes are more beneficial.

A further study completed by Gawler (2007)[3] states the following:

> In a 1998 study out of 10,661 women who were diagnosed with breast cancer, 4,638 were considered eligible for chemotherapy. From this

group only 164 gained some survival benefit, i.e., chemotherapy increased five year survival in early breast cancer by 3.5 percent.

The aim of the great majority of chemotherapy is palliative, not curative. This being so, the question then becomes: What is the most effective form of palliation and, in individual cases, do the side effects of chemotherapy warrant its use in palliative treatment?

Gawler also quotes from a study by Professor G Jelinek of Sir Charles Gairdner Hospital, Perth which states:

Chemotherapy is mainly palliative and not necessarily curative. People with advanced cancer are more willing to accept chemotherapy with a lower chance and a shorter duration of benefit than others imagine. Health professionals must recognise this when discussing treatment options with patients.

An article by an oncologist Eva Segelov (2006)[4], *The emperor's new clothes - can chemotherapy survive?* states:

Individual patients are concerned about their own chance of survival. Many patients will accept chemotherapy despite the small absolute benefit in survival.

Research by Duric et al. (2005)[5] on women who had received chemo for a period of three months, for early stage breast cancer revealed that 50 percent would have one more round of chemotherapy, even if it were to add only one more day to a promised five-year survival rate.

I found the study done by Cancer Treatment Centers of America (CTCA®) and Surveillance, Epidemiology and End Results (SEER) in 2017 and added their chart below for your information.

The chart of patient survival rate, plotted over 5 years from the CTCA and SEER databases, as shown in figure 1, reflects the survival rates of patients who were diagnosed and/or partially treated at a CTCA or SEER hospital. All patients included in the study were diagnosed between the year 2000 and 2013 with distant (metastatic) breast cancer. It includes estimates of the percentage of breast cancer patients with distant (metastatic) disease who survived for six months to five years after the initial diagnosis, as recorded in the CTCA and SEER databases.

CTCA and SEER patient survival rates

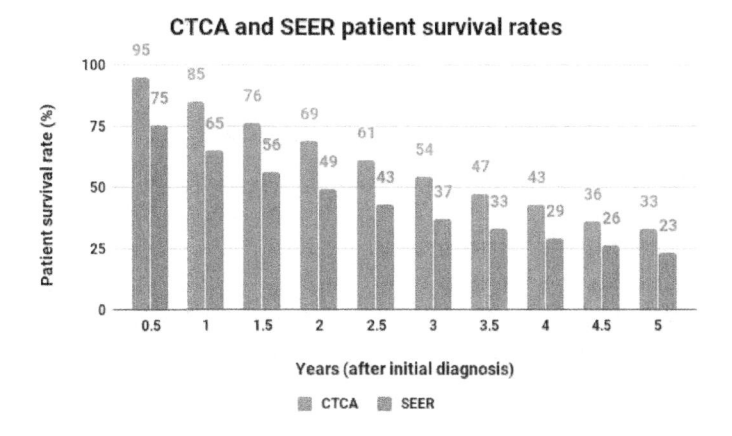

Years	CTCA	SEER
0.5	95	75
1	85	65
1.5	76	56
2	69	49
2.5	61	43
3	54	37
3.5	47	33
4	43	29
4.5	36	26
5	33	23

Fig. 1 Patient survival rates from Cancer Treatment Centres of America, comparing their statistics with the Surveillance, Epidemiology, and End Results (SEER) Program of the National Cancer Institute.[6]

Even though the 5 year survival rate has increased to between 23% and 33% compared to the 2.3% found in the Morgan, Ward and Barton study I would still not choose chemotherapy as my choice of treatment considering all the side effects (as listed below) which will limit the quality of one's life.

B. Side Effects

A further factor that I considered before deciding whether I would undergo chemotherapy was the possible side effects from the treatment itself.

The American Cancer Society list the possible side effects of chemotherapy for breast cancer as follows:[7]

26

- Hair loss
- Nail changes
- Mouth sores
- Loss of appetite or increased appetite
- Nausea and vomiting
- Diarrhoea
- Nerve damage (neuropathy)
- Hand-foot syndrome
- Chemo brain
- Feeling unwell or tired (fatigue)
- Heart damage
- Menstrual changes and fertility issues
- Increased risk of leukaemia
- You can also have sleep problems
- Some women also become depressed.
- Many drugs used to treat breast cancer, including the taxanes (docetaxel and paclitaxel), platinum agents (carboplatin, cisplatin), vinorelbine, eribulin and ixabepilone, can damage nerves outside of the brain and spinal cord. This can sometimes lead to symptoms (mainly in the hands and feet) like numbness, pain, burning or tingling sensations, sensitivity to cold or heat, or weakness.
- Many women who are treated for breast cancer report a slight decrease in mental functioning. They may have some problems with concentration and memory.
- Doxorubicin, epirubicin, and other chemotherapy drugs may cause permanent

heart damage (called cardiomyopathy).
- Effects on the blood-forming cells of the bone marrow, which can lead to increased chance of infections (from low white blood cell counts), easy bruising or bleeding (from low blood platelet counts), fatigue (from low red blood cell counts and other reasons) and various other possible side effects.
- For younger women, changes in menstrual periods are common side effects of chemotherapy. Premature menopause and infertility (not being able to fall pregnant) may occur and may be permanent.
- Very rarely certain chemotherapy drugs can cause diseases of the bone marrow, such as myelodysplastic syndrome or even acute myeloid leukemia, a cancer of white blood cells.

You can read more about these side effects on the American Cancer Society website.[7]

My mother had had chemotherapy for ovarian cancer a few years earlier. She personally experienced many of the side effects as listed above. For her, the experience was so difficult that she decided that she would never undergo any form of chemotherapy ever again. She fully supported my decision to go with the natural option.

C. Cancer Stem Cells Survive Radiation and Chemotherapy

These research articles were only released after I had already made my decision not to undergo chemotherapy, but I felt that they justified my decision so I included them in this book.

Researchers with the UCLA Department of Radiation Oncology, at UCLA's Jonsson Comprehensive Cancer Center, reported the results of a study they had carried out titled, Radiation Generates Cancer Stem Cells from Less Aggressive Breast Cancer Cells. (February 2012)[8] They concluded that radiation treatment (despite killing half of all tumour cells during every treatment) transforms other cancer cells into treatment-resistant breast cancer stem cells.

Pajonk, a scientist with the Eli and Edythe Broad Center of Regenerative Medicine at UCLA, states:
> We found that these induced breast cancer stem cells (iBCSC) were generated by radiation-induced activation of the same cellular pathways used to reprogram normal cells into induced pluripotent stem cells (iPS) in regenerative medicine. It was remarkable that these breast cancers used the same reprogramming pathways to fight back against the radiation treatment.

The article further states:

Breast cancer stem cells, thought to be the sole source of tumour recurrence, are known to be resistant to radiation therapy and don't respond well to chemotherapy.

The team also found that the iBCSC had a more than 30-fold increased ability to form tumors, compared with the non-irradiated breast cancer cells from which they originated. Pajonk says:

> The study unites the competing models of clonal evolution and the hierarchical organization of breast cancers, as it suggests that undisturbed, growing tumors maintain a small number of cancer stem cells. However, if challenged by various stressors that threaten their numbers, including ionizing radiation, the breast cancer cells generate iBCSC that may, together with the surviving cancer stem cells, repopulate the tumor.

An article from the John Hopkins Institute, titled, *Scientists Identify Chain Reaction That Shields Breast Cancer Stem Cells From Chemotherapy* (February 22, 2017)[9] states:

> Working with human breast cancer cells and mice, researchers at Johns Hopkins say they have identified a biochemical pathway that triggers the regrowth of breast cancer stem cells after chemotherapy. The regrowth of cancer stem cells is responsible for the drug resistance that develops in many breast tumors and the reason that for many patients, the

benefits of chemo are short-lived. Cancer recurrence after chemotherapy is frequently fatal.

Deciding that I would not do the chemotherapy I knew I was embarking on a road far less travelled. I will go on to describe each element of treatment I used in detail in the next chapters.

5. High-Dose Intravenous Vitamin C– My Primary Treatment.

I posed myself the following question: "If I only had another five years to live, would I rather live those years suffering from the side effects of chemotherapy and radiation, or would I prefer to function with vitality during those years by utilizing natural, alternate protocols?"

The diagnosis of breast cancer was a definite sign to me that my immune system wasn't operating at its optimum. Therefore, it made more sense to me to use therapies that would assist the immune system to recover, instead of compromising it even further. I decided to use high-dose intravenous vitamin C as one of the therapies to eliminate the breast cancer.

I was choosing the healing road less travelled, especially in South Africa, where I live. Here, conventional treatment of cancer is the way that is predominantly practised. Following a natural way to heal cancer would undoubtedly bring me resistance, scepticism and criticism.

However, I would never look back on following this path with any form of regret.

My friend Suret Morkel (microbiologist, medical scientist and natural practitioner) had been

administering high-dose Vitamin C intravenous (IVC) drips, with no side effects, at her practice. She treated various ailments, among them cancer, and encouraged me with her knowledge. Suret said:
> I even saw cancer healed within two weeks, on high dose IVC (50mg/ml up to 75mg/ml per drip). This is due to the high dose of Vitamin C (ascorbate) delivering peroxide, that in sick cells do the healing, yet do not affect healthy cells. It is similar to when you put a drop of peroxide on your skin-where the skin is intact nothing happens, but where there is a sore on the skin, it will bubble and eventually heal the sore.

A short historical background of high-dose vitamin C therapy:

I have included some technical information, as I believe here it is essential to establish and clarify a scientific basis to underscore such an important decision.

The first piece of research I list is an article taken from the *International Journal of Cancer Research*. (Ohno, Ohno, Suzuki, Gen-Ichiro& Inoue, 2008)[1] :
> Vitamin C (ascorbic acid or ascorbate) is one of the early unorthodox therapies for cancer, based on two hypotheses. Nearly 50 years ago, McCormick postulated that ascorbate protects against cancer by increasing collagen synthesis.

In 1972, Cameron and Rotman hypothesized that ascorbate could have anti-cancer action by inhibiting hyaluronidase and thereby preventing cancer spread. These hypotheses were subsequently popularized by Cameron and Pauling. They published case reports of 50 patients, some of whom seemed to have benefited from high-dose intravenous (IVC) ascorbate treatment.

The article also refers to a stage when vitamin C was, however, brought into question as a suitable treatment for cancer by a Mayo Clinic study in which randomized clinical trials, conducted with oral ascorbate alone, showed no benefit (Creagan et al., 1979)[2]. It then refers to a study by Chen et al (2005)[3,4]:

> Consequently, Chen et al suggested that ascorbic acid at pharmacological concentrations, only achievable with IVC, in the blood may be a pro-drug for H_2O_2 delivery to tissues, with major therapeutic implications. If unambiguous benefit can be shown even in a few cases, the use of ascorbic acid should be explored in more controlled studies. After all, even a small benefit is worthwhile as ascorbic acid is non-toxic and inexpensive, in contrast to the many chemotherapeutic agents in use. If the results show a clear lack of benefit, the use of ascorbic acid as a chemotherapeutic agent in cancer should be abandoned.

Another person who researched vitamin C was Dr Linus Carl Pauling (1901-1994), a physical chemist and peace activist who won two Nobel Prize awards, one in chemistry in 1954, followed by a Nobel Peace Prize in 1962. He introduced high doses of Vitamin C to fight many diseases, including cancer.

He believed that vitamin C has a pro-oxidant effect on cancer cells, and that it could assist in detoxifying diverse toxins present in a human body, such as carbon monoxide, alcohol, drugs, pesticides, radiation, heavy metals, mushroom toxins and even snake and spider venom. These studies are discussed and carefully recorded in his book, *How to Live Longer and Feel Better - Even With Cancer*, (1986)[5] and provided some evidence of the effectiveness of intravenously administered vitamin C.

The third researcher I would like to mention is Dr Hugh Riordan. His clinic produced more conclusive evidence than Dr Pauling. Dr Riordan conducted research on intravenous vitamin C for cancer patients. He discovered that vitamin C can be safely administered by intravenous infusion at maximum doses of one hundred grams or less, provided the precautions outlined in his protocol were taken.

He also found that, due to a deficiency in vitamin C in those with cancer, if large amounts of vitamin

C are presented to cancer cells, large amounts will be absorbed.

Because cancer cells are relatively low in an intracellular anti-oxidant enzyme called catalase, the high dose vitamin C induction of peroxide will continue to build up until it eventually causes dissolution of the cancer cell from the inside out. This effectively makes high-dose IVC a non-toxic chemotherapeutic agent.

Dr Riordan was able to prove that Vitamin C was selectively toxic to cancer cells if given intravenously. On the issue of vitamin C and cancer he concluded that: There are several potential benefits to giving IVC to cancer patients. (Riordan, Riordan, Meng & Jackson, 1995)[6]
- He discovered that, in sufficient concentrations, vitamin C could also kill viruses, bacteria and other germs. It could also cure chronic, systemic diseases like lupus and multiple sclerosis, and that all cancers responded well to high-dose vitamin C therapy without any side effects.
- Cancer patients are often depleted of vitamin C, and IVC provides an efficient means of restoring tissue stores.
- IVC has been shown to improve quality of life in cancer patients.
- IVC reduces inflammation (as measured by C - reactive protein levels) and reduces the production of pro-inflammatory cytokines.

- At high concentrations, ascorbate is preferentially toxic to tumour cells and an angiogenesis inhibitor.

The Riordan Clinic has treated hundreds of cancer patients (see figure 2 below) using the Riordan protocol. At the same time, the Riordan Clinic Research Institute (RCRI) has been researching the potential of intravenous vitamin C therapy for over thirty years. Their efforts have included in-vitro studies, animal studies, pharmacokinetic analyses, and clinical trials.

Types of cancers treated with IVC by the Riordan clinic

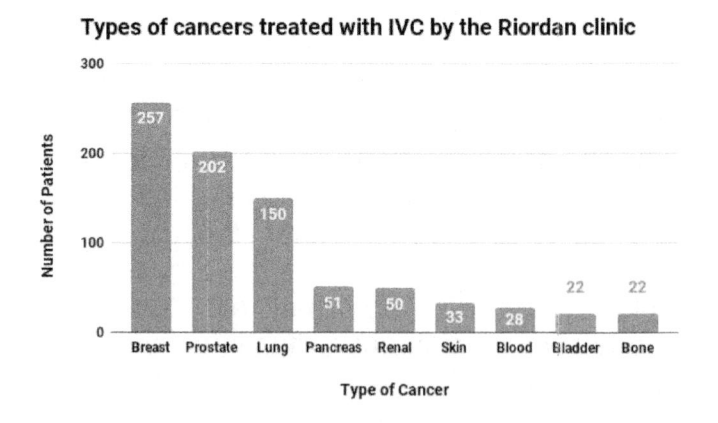

Type of Cancer	Number of Patients
Breast	257
Prostate	202
Lung	150
Pancreas	51
Renal	50
Skin	33
Blood	28
Bladder	22
Bone	22

Fig 2. Types of cancer treated with IVC by the Riordan clinic. (2013)[7].

The Riordan clinical trials concluded that "Vitamin C can accumulate in tumours, with significant tumour growth inhibition seen (in guinea pigs) at intra-tumour concentrations of 1 milliMolar (mM) or higher." (2013)[7]

You can find more about the Riordan report and protocols of actual dosage by reading the document from the Riordan Clinic Research Institute, titled *The Riordan IVC Protocol for Adjunctive Cancer Care Intravenous Ascorbate as a Chemotherapeutic and Biological Response Modifying Agent.* (2013)[7]

Further evidence of the effectiveness of intravenous vitamin C came to light after my decision, which confirmed to me that I had made the right choice.

In 2014 there was another study of the effectiveness of intravenous vitamin C, titled *Breast Cancer Patients - Treatment Choices and Outcomes in a Naturopathic Clinic* (Huber, NMD, FNORI Fellow, Naturopathic Oncology Research Institute, USA)[8]. The study states:

> Our clinic conducted a survey by questionnaire to breast cancer patients who had in common the following: a biopsy-diagnosed breast cancer, Stage I through late Stage IV, and that they stayed in our care for at least 4 treatments of IV nutrient infusions.

Those treatments involved sterile infusions of primarily, by volume and osmolarity, high-dose intravenous vitamin C (HDIVC), which has been studied in numerous venues for anti-cancer effect. Oral dosing of ascorbic acid has not been found to achieve sufficiently high concentrations in the vascular system to kill cancer cells.

However, intravenous use of ascorbic acid rose to plasma concentrations that were associated with apoptosis of cancer cells in vivo, and in vitro. Intravenous doses of ascorbic acid have been found to produce from 25 to 70 times as much plasma concentration as may be attained by oral administration.

The study goes on to say: ***HDIVC were found to kill cancer cells while leaving normal tissue unharmed.***

6. Treatment Protocols by an Integrated Health Professional

My first step of action was to make an appointment with a holistic integrative health practitioner to start off my healing journey. Dr Herman Spies was the integrative health practitioner of my choice. Bruce recovered remarkably under his treatment protocols. This while conventional doctors and dentists denied that mercury poisoning could occur from amalgam or the removal of it from teeth.

Dr Spies is registered with both the Health Professions Council of South Africa as a medical doctor, as well as the Allied Health Professions Council of South Africa for homoeopathy, acupuncture and as a doctor of Chinese medicine. (For more details about his practice, visit his website: www.drspies.com.)

A QUANTEC® scan, an original digital photograph of the patient's energy field, is taken at every visit to identify existing disorders at an electromagnetic level. The QUANTEC® scans more than 50 000 remedies in over 200 databases for a response.

The scans, being amazingly accurate, revealed that I needed to be treated for invasive intraductal breast cancer, malignant neoplasm of the lymph, lymph drainage problems, parasites, heavy metal toxicity (largely from amalgam fillings present at that time) and many digestive and hormonal imbalances and disorders.

My holistic treatment by Dr Spies involved the following modalities: High dose vitamin C drips, Electromagnetic Homeopathic solutions, supplements and herbs, footbaths, the use of the rife resonator machine and others. I go into the detail of each one below:

A. High-Dose Intravenous Vitamin C Drips

This was the main treatment I employed to rid my body of cancer cells. The drips are made up of a cocktail of high-dose intravenous Vitamin C (IVC) and small quantities of liquid magnesium, selenium, glutathione, manganese , zinc and B6.

Glutathione and selenium are important for detoxification, especially of heavy metals. The other ingredients provide important minerals to build up and support the immune system.

My protocol was as follows:
   Week 1: 1 x 15 g infusion per day, 2-3 per week.
   Week 2: 1 x 30 g infusion per day, 2-3 per week.
   Week 3: 1 x 65 g infusion per day, 2-3 per week.
   Week 4: 1 x 65 g infusion per day, 2-3 per week.

The high dose of vitamin C (65g) was given in a drip bag of 1000ml saline solution administered over 60 minutes per infusion.

The treatment was tapered down after the four-week intensive treatment until it was only necessary to do one 65g infusion once a month.

I experienced no dehabilitating side effects and could continue with my day-to-day living as normal.

It is, however, important to administer the IVC cocktail slowly - at least 60 minutes per infusion. I did find that if it was done in a shorter time frame, I would feel queasy afterwards for about an hour.

I continued to have the high-dose vitamin C drips once a month for a further two years.

B.   Electromagnetic   Homeopathic Solutions

The electromagnetic homeopathic drops were produced through analysing the relevant frequencies of the person on the day of the QUANTEC® scan. The QUANTEC® scan generates a healing recipe, unique to each patient, containing all the relevant frequencies needed to correct the existing dysfunction at the electromagnetic level.

Electromagnetic Homeopathic Mixes assist in:
- **Killing parasites:** Parasites can cause major damage to the human body, weakening the immune system and in turn causing disease.

The Bilharzia parasite was identified as the main parasite in my body. Dr Spies mentioned that this could have contributed to the breast cancer.
- **Detoxifying from metals and toxins:** We are exposed to heavy metals and toxins daily through the air we breathe, water we drink, food we eat and especially amalgam fillings in our mouths. Detoxification from these is vitally important to allow the immune system to recover and in turn heal the cancer.
- **Restoring the cells:** The health of cells is important to their orderly growth.
- **Glandular and organ support:** Specific electromagnetic homeopathic drops supported my adrenals, thyroid, heart, colon and other organs.
- **Ridding the body of candida:** The drops help to get rid of yeast and candida. Candida is a fungal growth that can penetrate the intestinal wall and allow small particles of food directly into the bloodstream, a condition called leaky gut, resulting in allergies and a host of other symptoms.

C. Supplements and Herbs

I used the following supplements and herbs:
- **Boswellia (Frankincense)** to fight inflammation. It is well known that inflammation is one of the main causes of cancer. I loved the smell of the Boswellia

tablets. I felt like my body was agreeing that this was the correct medicine for it.
- **Sutherlandia**, a powerful immune booster. Sutherlandia is also called the cancerbush or kankerbos. Cancerbush is regarded as the most significant and multi-purposed of the medicinal plants in Southern Africa. It powerfully assists the body to mobilize its own resources to cope with physical and mental stresses. It is therefore an adaptogen in the class of herbs such as astragalus, ginseng and ashwagandha, and has even been referred to as African ginseng. This can be taken as a tea or in tablet form. The tea, however, is extremely bitter so I preferred it in tablet form.
- **Omega 3** to help fight inflammation. I took fish oil tablets in gel capsule form-one gram per day. You need to make sure you get fish oil that is free from heavy metals, especially mercury - which is present in a number of fish nowadays. Generally, the larger the fish and the further up the feeding chain, the more mercury is present in it. Mercury is the second most toxic metal to us as humans and can cause havoc to the immune system.
- **Neurest,** a natural mood and immune enhancer, this tablet is produced by Suret Morkel at Innerfruits. It contains DL phenylanine, Vitamins B1, B6 and B12, magnesium, calcium, chromium, l-glutamine, MSM and folic acid. I took at least two of these per day. It helped me to stay calm and stress-

free. I still take one tablet per day to keep my stress levels under control.
- **Melatonin** to help with sleep. Melatonin, also known as N-acetyl-5-methoxy tryptamine, is a hormone that is produced by the pineal gland and regulates sleep and wakefulness. Melatonin tablets provide a bit more of this naturally-produced hormone to induce sleep. Sleep is considered the most important process to restore and heal the body.
- **Probiotics** to help with digestion and restoration of the gut flora. A healthy gut is important for bolstering the immune system. See the section on the "The Gut and Cancer", Chapter 8, where the gut is discussed in some detail.
- **Digestive enzymes** to help with digestion. If we don't have enough digestive enzymes, we can't break down our food, which means that even though we're eating well, we aren't absorbing all the good nutrition. Low-grade inflammation in the digestive tract can be caused by food allergies, intestinal permeability, parasitic infection and so on. This can lead to deficiencies in digestive enzymes. Low stomach acid levels and chronic stress results in a constant state of fight-or-flight, which can cause impaired digestive enzyme output.
- **Tissue salts** to restore mineral balance. Tissue salts, also known as cell salts or biochemistry salts, are the same minerals

found in rocks and soil. They naturally occur in the human body, which means that an imbalance or lack of certain salts opens the door to illness and disease. The intention was to balance my tissue salts.
- **Ultra InflamX** by Metagenics(Amipro) as a dietary food supplement. This rice protein-based formula is enhanced with L-glutamine* and a special phytonutrient blend of ginger, rosemary, turmeric** and green tea extract.

*L- glutamine supports intestinal mucosal cells and also helps with the production of glutathione, which assists in the detoxification of the liver.

**Turmeric has many cancer-fighting properties. Researchers have been studying the ingredient curcumin, found in turmeric, as a beneficial herb in cancer treatment. (Ravindran, Prasad & Aggarwal, 2009)[1]

It is important to check with your health practitioner on the dosage suitable for you and ensure there are no clashes with any other medications you might be taking.

D. Footbaths

Ionic footbaths are used for reducing the toxic load in the body. Dr Spies advocated these based on his study and qualification in Chinese medicine.

The Pacific College of Oriental Medicine's Pauline Adamo (2017)[2] states that:

"Most people can benefit from an ionic detox. It is especially good for those suffering from GI disorders, skin conditions, fungal or yeast infections, and cancer." She also says that "Other scientifically measured effects of this detox, besides alkalization, are lower blood sugar levels and lower cholesterol levels."

E. Rife Resonator Machine

Dr Spies is an advocate of the Rife Resonator machine. The machine was invented by Dr Rife in the 1930's. It could send out frequencies that hindered or destroyed the growth of certain cells. Initially the frequencies were limited but were later added to, as the machines were developed further.

The frequencies can be set to target parasites or specific types of cell growth, such as cancer cells. During a session on the Rife machine, the frequencies are programmed to change so as to expose the parasites and cells identified as unwanted in your body.

I used the machine for a number of months. For more information on the successes of doctors who used the machine, see the following website: *Your Rife Machine History Educational Website*.[3]

F. Other Protocols recommended by Dr Spies

- Lymphatic drainage via Air Therapy and

Ozone Saunas
- Dietary changes
- Emotional healing

I will discuss these in more depth in separate chapters.

7. My Cancer-Fighting Diet.

"Let food be thy medicine and medicine be thy food."
Hippocrates, father of medicine, in 431 B.C.

It is not only the way that we eat today but also what we ate in our recent and even less recent past that can harm our immune system. These habits can make us more susceptible to cancer in our later lives.

The food you eat today influences what happens to your health in the future.

My diet was less than desirable from the age of 19, until I got married at the age of 33. I didn't make myself nutritious food at home, ate mainly buffet canteen food for lunch, and restaurant food at night. Sometimes I would still my hunger with two chocolates for lunch (an unthinkable act now). At home I mostly ate bread, cereals, flavoured yogurts and cheese, with some fruit but no green vegetables. My diet consisted mainly of refined carbohydrates and processed foods.

The results of this nutritionally-poor diet did show up in my health. I started to experience constipation at the age of 24. This I solved by adding wheat bran to my tea in the mornings. I was totally unaware that the wheat bran could irritate the intestinal lining and lead to leaky gut, overgrowth of intestinal bacteria and malabsorption of nutrients.

One of the first nutrient deficiencies that showed up was that of iron. I became very anaemic, not immediately evident, as my menstruation remained normal. A doctor even did a colonoscopy to find out why I was so anaemic. Nothing was picked up and he prescribed iron supplements. Diet was never discussed.

If my diet had been correctly analysed and a holistic approach applied, this situation could have been rectified. Adding red meat to my diet, even once a week, would have supplied some of my iron requirements. Legumes and green, leafy vegetables for the rest of the week, would have supplied the remainder.

The severe eczema I suffered from in my thirties was another manifestation of my poor diet, which had led to a leaky gut, poor absorption of nutrients and therefore many allergies. Restoring the gut would have helped a lot to resolve this. I explain the gut and its importance in some detail in the next chapter.

A. Why I Chose a Vegan Diet

Once diagnosed with cancer, I was determined to live and get well. I was prepared to make drastic changes to my lifestyle. My existing diet had already undergone some adjustments. I had removed sugar, gluten and milk, and included more fruit and vegetables, to try and resolve the eczema that plagued me. However, I learned that there was still much room for improvement.

A friend of mine, Colleen, gave me an audio version of a book called *The China Study, The Most Comprehensive Study of Nutrition Ever Conducted and the Startling Implications for Diet, Weight Loss, and Long-term Health*. Thomas Campbell, T. Colin Campbell (2006). Among many other subjects, it covers the well-documented cancer-protective and cancer-inhibitive factors in fruits and vegetables and the negative effect of a high animal-protein diet.

I decided to go on a completely vegan diet, which I followed for almost 2 years after my diagnosis. I would highly recommend a vegan diet to anyone who wants to heal cancer naturally. For this diet to be effective it needs to be followed for at least six months.

Three main Reasons for a Vegan Diet at the Start of the Healing Journey.

I. IGF-1 Levels in Animal Products

The main reason for eliminating animal products (including beef, lamb, pork, chicken, fish, eggs and dairy) for the first six months, is that all animal products contain IGF-1 (insulin-like growth factor 1). This compound has been found to stimulate tumour growth, especially in breast and prostate cancer.

A study published by NCBI, *The Role of the Insulin-like Growth Factor-1 System in Breast Cancer* (Christopoulos, Msaouel & Koutsilieris, 2015)[1] found:
> A growing body of evidence points to the important role of the IGF-1 system in breast cancer development, progression and metastasis. IGF-1 is a point of convergence for major signalling pathways implicated in breast cancer growth.

A review of 17 studies found that IGF-1 is positively associated with breast cancer risk. This takes levels of IGF binding protein 3 into account, owing to its effects on oestrogen-sensitive tumours. (Appleby, Reeves & Roddam, 2010)[2]

Does IGF-1 Cause Cancer?

The short answer to this is no. IGF-1 doesn't cause cancer, though it may allow cancerous cells that already exist to grow faster. If you are diagnosed with breast cancer or prostate cancer, it may be appropriate to take steps towards lowering IGF-1 levels. (Rigby, n.d.)[3]

II.   Methionine in Animal products.
Methionine is an essential amino acid in the human diet. Animal products are high in methionine, and it has been proven in a number of

studies that methionine is required for tumours to grow. Here are the conclusions of just three such studies:

- Many human cancer cell lines and primary tumours have absolute requirements for methionine. In contrast, normal cells are relatively resistant to exogenous methionine restriction. (Cellarier et al., 2003)[4]
- Methionine restriction (best achieved through a plant-based diet) may prove to have a major impact on patients with cancer because, unlike normal tissues, many human tumours require the amino acid methionine to grow. (Greger, 2013)[5]
- There is direct evidence that methionine restriction leads to selective death of cancer cells. In a study on targeting tumour initiating cells, researchers conclude that the inhibition of protein synthesis is a new therapeutic strategy for eradicating these cells. (Lamb et al., 2015)[6]

Methionine-containing foods include beef, lamb, cheese, turkey, pork, fish, shellfish, soy, eggs, dairy, nuts and beans. The bioavailability of methionine is greater in animal foods, particularly dairy, than in beans and nuts. (Whitbread, 2018)[7]

III. Food Transit Time (mouth to bowel movement)

The longer the transit time from mouth to bowel movement, the more a food affects our immune system and the healing process negatively. Animal products can slow the transit time as proved in the studies below.

According to a study published in the *British Journal of Nutrition*, Gear, Brodribb, Ware & Mannt, (1981)[8]:
> The average transit time for a vegetarian group was nearly 24 hours faster than for non-vegetarians. The researchers attributed the difference in transit times between vegetarians and meat-eaters to the amount of fibre in the diet. Vegetarians consume more fibre than meat-eaters, because plant-based foods make up a greater part of the vegetarian diet. Animal protein also contains more fat, which requires longer periods to digest than carbohydrates.

The below conclusions are based on a study by Dr Wjatscheslaw Wlassoff (2015)[9]:
> A bowel transit time of more than two days increases the risk of weakening the overall immune system. A long transit time means toxins and wastes are re-circulating back to the blood stream, resulting in fatigue, headaches, acne, allergies, muscle pain, joint pains, gas, bloating and other symptoms.

A study done by the National Food Institute of the Technical University of Denmark as cited in *Nutrition Insight*, (2016)[10] found that:

The longer food takes to pass through the colon, the more harmful bacteria degradation products are produced. Tine Rask Licht explains that "When the transit time is shorter, we find a higher amount of the substances that are produced to renew the colon's inner surface which could lead to a healthier intestinal wall."

You can help the transit time by eating a diet high in fibre and by limiting the intake of meat. You should also drink more water.

B. Cancer -Fighting Foods
I. Cruciferous Vegetables

There is no other vegetable group that has so many cancer-fighting components as these vegetables. They are an absolute must in any cancer-fighting and preventative diet. This food group is still part of my diet today, because of its incredible anti-cancer benefits.

Among this group of vegetables are:
- Arugula
- Bok Choy
- Broccoli
- Brussels sprouts
- Cabbage
- Cauliflower
- Chinese cabbage
- Collard greens

- Horseradish
- Kale
- Mustard greens
- Radish
- Shepherd's purse
- Turnip
- Watercress

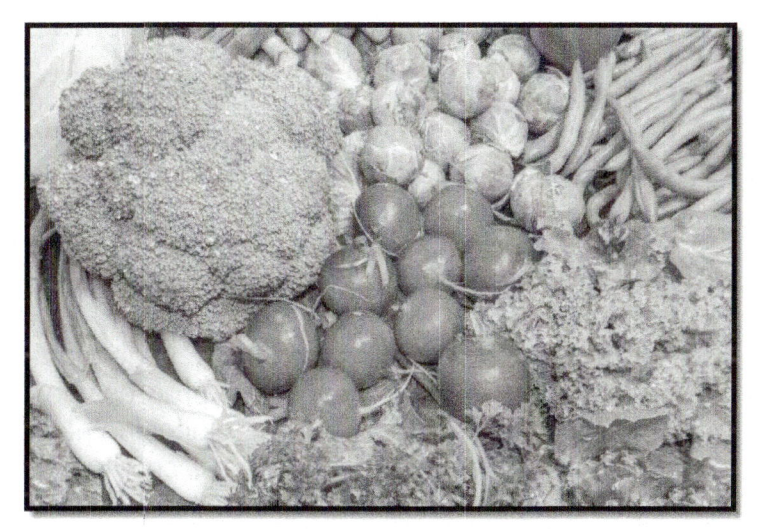

Fig. 3 Examples of cruciferous vegetables.

The following are Cancer-fighting Components present in Cruciferous Vegetables (NCI 2012)[11]:
- **Sulfurophane:** Researchers have found that sulfurophane induces phase-2 enzymes that detoxify carcinogens. In addition, sulfurophane induces apoptosis, inhibits NF-kB and scavenges free radicals, thereby helping block

cancer cell growth. (Anand et al., 2008; Watson, Beaver, Williams, Dashwood & Ho, 2013)[12,13]

- **Indole-3-carbinol:** Researchers suspect indole-3-carbinol is one of several vegetable components that might protect against cancer. A study conducted in 2008 (Weng, Tsai, Kulp, & Chen)[14] states: "Moreover, indole-3-carbinol proves to be an effective chemo preventive agent against estrogen-responsive cancers such as breast and cervical cancers. This broad spectrum of antitumor activities in conjunction with low toxicity underscores the translational value of indole-3-carbinol and its metabolites in cancer prevention/therapy." A further study regarding indole-3-carbinol (Royston & Tollefsboll, 2015)[15] says the following: "There is more than just one mechanism by which cruciferous vegetables negatively impact cancer progression." Indoles, another derivative of glucosinolates, are found in abundance in cruciferous vegetables, and indole-3-carbinol is showing promising evidence as a cancer preventive therapeutic.
- **Phytochemicals:** Regular consumption of cruciferous vegetables leads to high intake of unusual phytochemicals known as glucosinolates and consequently exposure of cells to isothiocyanates. Isothiocyanates are well-known protectors against carcinogenesis and modulators of the activities of enzymes

involved in the metabolism of carcinogens, especially by the induction of phase 2 detoxication enzymes. Glucosinolates and their isothiocyanate hydrolysis products are well-known protectors against carcinogenesis. (Talaley & Fahey, 2001)[16]
- **Fibre:** Cruciferous vegetables are a good source of fibre. A study (Vineetha, 2014)[17] has revealed that consuming 30 grams of soluble and insoluble fibre per day can reduce the risk of breast cancer. It also reduces the risk of ovarian cancer by almost 20 percent. Dietary fibre, also known as roughage, is a nutrient required for proper digestion of food. Besides assisting with smooth bowel movements, fibre can also reduce the risk of heart disease, stroke and hypertension.
- **Cruciferous vegetables are high in soluble as well as insoluble fibre.** One cup of steamed broccoli can provide you with 5.1 grams of fibre. Brussels sprouts can contribute 4.1 grams of fibre to your body. Cabbage can help you meet 12 percent of the daily amount of fibre. Kale contains four grams of fibre per cup. One cup of cauliflower provides you with two grams of fibre.

Cruciferous vegetables also provide a variety of other nutrients as shown in table 1 below:

Nutrient	Broccoli	Brussels Sprouts	Cabbage	Collard Greens

	Steamed	Boiled	Boiled	Boiled
Vitamin A (IU)	5178	1840	600	12008
Vitamin B1 (mg)	0.20	0.28	0.27	0.16
Vitamin B2 (mg)	0.41	0.20	0.24	0.40
Vitamin B3 (mg)	2.13	1.56	1.27	2.20
Vitamin B6 (mg)	0.50	0.46	0.52	0.48
Folic Acid (mcg)	213	154	91	357
Vit C (mg)	279	159	91	70
Vit E (mg)	1.70	2.18	0.70	3.37
Vit K (mcg)	351	359	221	1422
Iron (mg)	3.1	3.1	0.79	1.76
Magnesium (mg)	88	51	36	65
Manganese (mg)	0.77	0.57	0.55	2.16
Phosphorous (mg)	234	143	68	100
Potassium (mg)	1146	810	439	998
Zinc (mg)	1.41	0.51	0.42	1.62
Protein (g)	10.6	6.5	4.6	9.5
Fiber (g)	10.6	6.7	10.5	10.7
Omega-3 fatty acids (g)	0.45	0.43	0.52	0.36

Table 1. A summary of the nutrient richness of cruciferous vegetables: (The Healthiest Foods website, 2018)[18]. Amount for each vegetable is a 100 calories.

It is difficult to find another vegetable group that is as high in vitamin A (carotenoids), vitamin C, folic acid and fibre as the cruciferous vegetables.
Kale and collards are also high in vitamin K.

Vitamin K helps regulate our inflammatory response, including chronic, excessive inflammatory responses that can increase our risk of cancer.

Cruciferous vegetables contribute a surprising amount of protein-over 25 percent of the daily requirement in three cups.

Many B-complex vitamins are concentrated in cruciferous vegetables, as are certain minerals.

This food group also contains its own unique set of phytonutrients - the glucosinolates - that are simply unavailable to the same extent in any other food group.

Cooking of Cruciferous Vegetables.

Cruciferous vegetables are best steamed or cooked in soups or stews. Eating them raw in large amounts can inhibit thyroid hormones, which are vital for the functioning of the body. The insoluble fibre (between one and two grams in half a cup of cruciferous vegetables) makes them hard to digest when eaten raw. But by cooking these vegetables we lose most of the enzyme breakdown products.

Dr Michael Greger, MD.FACLM (2016)[19] wrote the following in an article called *How to Cook Broccoli*:
> There is a strategy to get the benefits of raw in cooked form. In raw broccoli, the sulforaphane precursor, called glucoraphanin, mixes with the enzyme (myrosinase) when you chew or chop it. If given enough time - such as when sitting in

your upper stomach waiting to get digested-sulforaphane is born. The precursor and sulforaphane are resistant to heat and therefore cooking, but the enzyme is destroyed. No enzyme = no sulforaphane. That's why I described the "hack and hold" technique-if we chop the broccoli, brussels sprouts, kale, collards, or cauliflower first and then wait 40 minutes, we can cook them all we want. The sulforaphane is already made; the enzyme has already done its job, so we don't need it anymore.

Another beneficial way to eat cruciferous vegetables raw is by eating them fermented. Not only are fermented vegetables full of beneficial bacteria for the gut but are easily digestible . Sauerkraut is a good option for eating raw cabbage.

II. Berries.

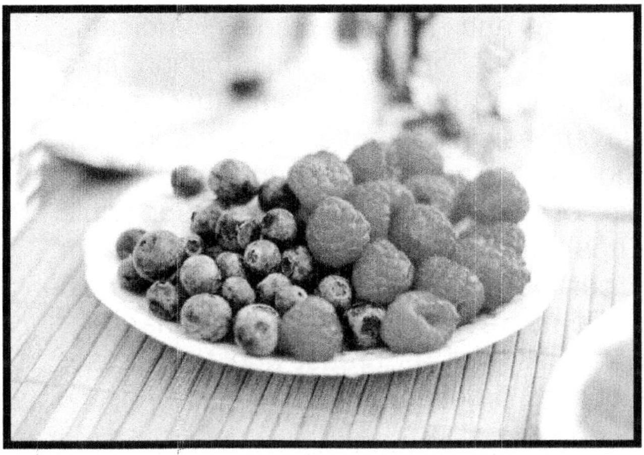

Fig. 4 Delicious, nutritious berries.

I don't know about you, but I love something sweet in my diet. The abundant variations of sweetness found in different types of berries are a wonderful option to include in any diet.

Berries are not only delicious, but also contain some powerful cancer-fighting qualities. Strawberries, blueberries, cranberries, raspberries and blackberries hide a nutritional secret that could help to avoid chronic disease, including cancer.

Studies have found that diets marked by high consumption of berries are inhibitory to many forms of cancer. An extensive study (Kristo, Klimis

Zacas & Sikalidis, 2016)[20] came to the following conclusion:

> The work we have summarized herein, primarily from in vivo and human studies, indicates favourable effects of berry consumption in a variety of cancers by mechanisms that involve oxidative stress, inflammation and the related signalling. It appears rather doubtful that a particular compound in berries is responsible for the health benefits these food items extend. Edible berries have been demonstrated to extend chemoprevention in cancer primarily of the GI tract as well as breast and to a lesser degree of liver, prostate, pancreas and lung.

Fresh Berries Anti-Cancer Facts:
Below are some of the nutritional components of fresh berries that can be cancer inhibiting. (Berry Health Benefits Network, n.d.)[21]

- **Anthocyanins:** These colour pigments in berries are powerful antioxidants. Blue, purple and red colours have been associated with a lower risk for cancer.
- **Antioxidants:** These are substances that protect the body by neutralizing free radicals or unstable oxygen molecules, which can damage the cells and are a major cause of disease and aging.
- **Phytochemicals:** Phytochemicals are naturally occurring antioxidants in plants that add flavour, colour pigments and scent; they are abundant in all types of fruits and

vegetables, particularly berries.
- **Catechins:** Catechins are flavonols* that support the antioxidant defence system. Catechins found in raspberries and blackberries are very similar to those found in green tea, which studies show may contribute to cancer prevention. The catechin content found in 100 grams of raspberries berries is a whopping 83 milligrams (the highest of all the berries) . * Flavonols are just one of many groups of phytochemicals.
- **Dietary Fibre:** Fibre helps maintain a healthy GI tract, lowers blood cholesterol, reduces heart disease and may prevent cancer.
- **Ellagic Acid:** Scientists believe that ellagic acid plays a major role in cancer prevention and tumour reversal. These compounds work in synergy to both inhibit the growth of pre-malignant cancer cells and trigger the programmed death of cancer cells through apoptosis (Apoptosis is a type of cell death in which a series of molecular steps in a cell lead to its death. The process of apoptosis may be blocked in cancer cells).
- **Gallic Acid:** A potent antioxidant also found in black tea and red wine, gallic acid has been shown in tests (Russell et al., 2012)[22] to inhibit cell proliferation and cause cell death in cancer cells.
- **Quercetin:** This is a flavonol that works as both an anti-carcinogen and antioxidant; it also protects against cancer and heart disease.

- **Rutin:** A bioflavonoid that promotes vascular health, rutin helps to prevent cell proliferation associated with cancer, and has anti-inflammatory and anti-allergenic properties.
- **Salicylic Acid:** The salicylic acid found in blackberries and raspberries is proven to have the same protective effect against heart disease as aspirin. A 100g serving of red raspberries contains around 5mg of salicylic acid.
- **Vitamin C:** Vitamin C is a powerful antioxidant and helps protect against cancers, heart disease and stress. Vitamin C also helps in maintaining a healthy immune system, aids in neutralizing pollutants, is needed for antibody production and acts to increase the absorption of nutrients. Below is a short list of berries containing the highest concentration of vitamin C.

Indian gooseberry (Amla)	445 mg/100g
Strawberries:	57 mg/ 100g
Blackcurrants:	155 mg/100g
Redcurrants	58mg/100g
Raspberries:	32 mg/100g
Cape gooseberry	27.7mg/100g

I also love the Cape gooseberries that grow easily in the sandy soil of my garden. They are sweeter than Indian gooseberries (Amla) and a 100g serving can provide 27.7mg of vitamin C (46 percent of your daily vitamin C requirements).

Berries are a solid choice for one's anti-cancer food arsenal. I would recommend that 2-3 servings be eaten on a daily basis because of the incredible health benefits.

Just remember to buy organic berries, especially strawberries. Strawberries top this year's list of the produce with the highest level of pesticide residue, according to a new report from the Environmental Working Group (EWG). Nearly all of the non-organic strawberry samples (98 percent) had detectable pesticide residues. Some samples showed residue from 17 different pesticides. (Amarelo, 2017)[24]

III. Apricot Seed Kernels

An article titled *Apricot Seeds Kill Cancer Cells without Side Effects* (Fassa, 2009)[25] explains why I included apricot kernels into my daily diet:

> In 1952, Dr Ernest Krebb Jr, a biochemist in San Francisco, postulated that cancer could be a metabolic reaction to a poor diet, and that a missing nutrient from modern man's diet could be the key to overcoming cancer. His research led to a compound found in over 1,200 edible plants throughout nature.
>
> That compound is amagdylin, or vitamin B17. Apricot seed kernels contain the highest concentrations and necessary enzymes of amagdylin.

A primitive tribe, the Hunzas, were known to consume large amounts of apricot seed kernels. There was no incidence of cancer among them at all and they had long, healthy life spans.
There have been several testimonies from cancer victims who cured themselves by chewing large quantities of apricot seeds or kernels alone. Many practitioners and writers recommend you combine other alternative cancer therapies with the use of apricot pits.

I used it as an add-on to the other therapies that I used to overcome the cancer. I ate 3-5 pips a day, which I ground up with my flaxseed mix, and sprinkled over my breakfast and salads.

C. Juicing and Digestion

I wanted to ensure that every bite I took would be highly beneficial in rebuilding my body and contributing to my healing. My goal was to eliminate all foods that could be a burden to my body and only eat nutrient-dense food. I avoided ready-made meals and restaurant food, especially takeaway food. The latter especially are highly processed and full of sugar, preservatives, stabilizers and colorants.

The fresher the produce, the better it is for your body. Farmer's markets offer wonderful opportunities to buy super-fresh produce. I order my organic vegetables online from local farmers through www.thinkorganic.co.za.

Cancer patients almost always have difficulty digesting and absorbing food. This can be a result of toxicity, malfunction of the digestive system or a decrease in stomach acid production. My body was struggling to digest, assimilate and eliminate at an optimally-balanced rate, which resulted in periodic constipation, hay-fever, eczema and many mineral and vitamin deficiencies.

This is why juicing of vegetables and fruit is so highly effective at ensuring maximum absorption of nutrients.

Vegetable juicing formed an important part of my healing protocol, and one of the first things I included daily in my diet. The juice is considered already chewed, which ensures optimum digestion of nutrients from the food.

The Gerson® Therapy recommends 13 glasses of vegetable juice a day. Here is a quote from the Gerson Institute (2011)[25]:
This tremendous influx of liquids provides the nutritional equivalent of almost seventeen pounds of food a day. The consumption of that quantity of food on a daily basis would be impossible." (The Gerson Institute, 2011)[26]

Benefits of fruit and vegetable juicing

Dr Mercola, in an article in Waking Times (May 2003)27 lists some of the benefits of juicing:
- Juicing helps you absorb all the nutrients from the vegetables. This is important because most of us have impaired digestion.
- Juicing will help to pre-digest the food for you, so you will receive more of the nutritional value of the vegetables.
- Juicing allows you to consume an optimal amount of vegetables in an efficient manner.
- You can add a wider variety of vegetables in your diet. Many people eat the same vegetables and salads every day. But with juicing, you can juice a wide variety and quantity of vegetables that you may not normally enjoy or be capable of eating whole.
- Juicing increases your energy. You feel energized almost immediately, since the juice is in a more easily digestible state and can therefore be utilized by your body immediately.

Juicing also boosts your immune system with concentrated phytochemicals which can help revitalize your body.

Even if you are going through conventional chemotherapy treatment, vegetable juice will help you to recover more quickly from the harsh side effects.

My mom had chemotherapy for ovarian cancer and included juicing in her diet. The additional nutrients assisted her with more energy and she coped better with the severe side effects of the chemotherapy.

I made fresh vegetable juice daily and consumed at least 2-3 glasses per day. The vegetables that I found most palatable to drink were carrot, beetroot, spinach, cucumber and ginger, sweetened with organic apples or half a pineapple. I made the juice more palatable by diluting it down with water.

My favourite vegetable juice recipe:
(makes 4 glasses)
5-8 carrots
½ beet
2 spinach leaves or ½ cucumber or beet greens
5cm ginger root
1-2 organic apples or ½ pineapple

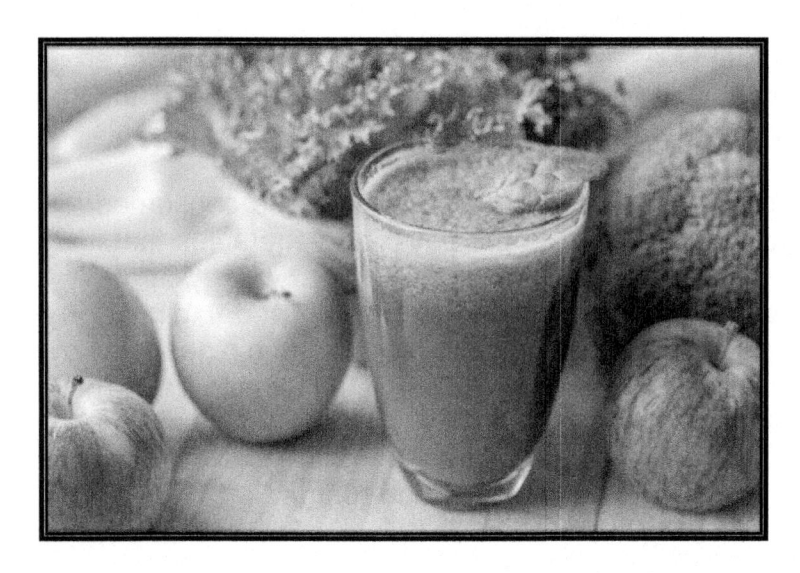

Just remember that vegetable juice is highly perishable; it's best to drink all of the freshly-made juice immediately. However, you can store it for up to 24 hours in the fridge (with minimal nutritional loss) by adding vitamin C.

D. Further Steps to Improve Digestion and Get the Nutrients You Need

Dr Susan E. Brown (2015)[28] mentions the following easy steps to improve digestion:
- Drink hot water and hot herbal teas. Both help detoxify the body and build digestive strength. Simmering a few slices of ginger root in boiling water makes a ginger root tea that stimulates digestion. Herbal teas of chamomile, peppermint and cinnamon also promote good digestion.

- Naturally fermented apple cider vinegar in half a glass of water before meals also promotes digestion.
- Eat and drink probiotic-rich foods. These include kefir (fermented milk), yogurt, sauerkraut, apple cider vinegar and kombucha
- Soak your beans, lentils and rice to enhance the fermentation process. Beans require a more lengthy period of soaking to lentils and rice.
- Chew your food well and eat at a moderate pace. Ideally, you should chew each mouthful some 30 times, breaking the food into small particles and allowing the salivary enzymes to begin their work of digesting the food.
- Eat in a peaceful and relaxed environment. If you do a little comparative test, you will note that you feel better and your digestion is smoother when you eat in a quiet, peaceful environment. Avoid watching television, reading, working, or arguing with others when you eat.
- Eat freshly-cooked foods. These are the most nourishing and are free of moulds or staleness. Don't eat leftovers if they have been standing for more than 24 hours.
- Avoid overeating. Excessive intake of food greatly burdens the entire digestive system. Practice moving away from the table while you are still a bit hungry.
- Eat cooked foods instead of cold or raw foods.

The eating of cooked food instead of cold or raw food is very much against the raw food movement. I couldn't understand why I didn't do well on a mostly raw diet at the start of my journey.

In traditional Ayurvedic medicine all cold and raw foods must be heated up to enhance digestion. People with weak digestion generally do well to eat little raw or cold food or drinks, and do better on hot soups, broths and casseroles.

E. Organic Fruits and Vegetables

Commercially-farmed vegetables are generally sprayed with toxic herbicides and pesticides. This increases the toxic load in the body and slows or even prevents the healing process. Pesticides are absorbed into the plants and fruit, so it's not effective to just wash a fruit or a vegetable.

Here are the 12 most toxic fruits and vegetables to avoid eating if they are not organic: apples, peaches, nectarines, strawberries, grapes, celery, spinach, sweet bell peppers, cucumbers, cherry tomatoes, snap peas and potatoes. (Oasis Integrative medicine 2017)[29]

The more toxins in the body, the more minerals and vitamins are needed by the body to help it to function at optimal levels and heal that which is out of balance.

Below are some pointers from a video, called *Why You Must Eliminate Pesticides in Food When Treating Cancer* (Bell, 2017),[30] on reasons to remove pesticides from food:

- Pesticides are endocrine disruptors. Some pesticides will destroy a hormone on contact. Others will mimic hormones.
- When we alter the endocrine function, we disrupt normal metabolic processes that keep us young, functioning and vital.
- As well as being endocrine disruptors, pesticides destroy the enzymes that are the essential tools of life.
- You cannot subsist on pesticide-laden foods and overcome cancer.

I tried to eat organic food as often as possible, to lower my toxic load. It is more expensive than commercially-farmed produce, but this was not the time for penny-pinching in this area.

It is important to eat food as soon as possible after cooking. Therefore store-bought, pre-made meals are not the best food to enhance your health, as there are certain bacteria that do survive the cold temperatures of the fridge. At a maximum, store food for one day in the fridge.

Never cover your food with plastic and heat it in a microwave. The heated plastic releases chemicals that enter your food, and these can act as endocrine disruptors. Endocrine disruptors can interfere with the hormonal systems, and this can cause cancerous tumours.

F. ORAC (Oxygen Radical Absorbance Capacity)

Studies now suggest that consuming fruits and vegetables with a high ORAC value may slow the aging process in both body and brain. ORAC values are a measure of antioxidant activity. Antioxidants inhibit oxidation (which is known to have a damaging effect on tissues). A diet of fruits and vegetables that allow you to consume between 3,000 and 5,000 ORAC units per day will help you maintain an optimal level of antioxidant protection from free radical damage.

Below is the ORAC Rating Table (Hammer Enterprises, 2009)[23]

Fruits	ORAC Value*	Vegetables	ORAC Value*
Açai Berry	18,500	Kale	1,770
Prunes	5,770	Spinach, raw	1,260
Raisins	2,830	Brussel Sprouts	980
Blueberries	2,400	Alfalfa Sprouts	930
Blackberries	2,036	Spinach, steamed	909
Cranberries	1,750	Broccoli	890

		Florets	
Strawberries	1,540	Beets	841
Pomegranates	1,245	Red Bell Pepper	713
Raspberries	1,220	Onion	450
Plums	949	Corn	400
Oranges	750	Eggplant	390
Red Grapes	739	Cauliflower	377
Cherries	670	Peas, frozen	364
Kiwifruit	602	White Potatoes	313
White Grapes	442	Sweet Potatoes	301
Cantaloupe	252	Carrots	207
Banana	221	String Beans	201
Apple	218	Tomatoes	189
Apricots	164	Zucchini	176
Peach	158	Yellow Squash	150

Table 2. ORAC ratings for various fruits and vegetables.
*ORAC value per 100 grams (approximately 3.5 ounces)

Antioxidants are shown to work best when eaten in wholesome, unprocessed food; the presence of fibre and other plant compounds enhance the health benefit.

G. My Typical Daily Vegan Menu

During my period as a vegan, which lasted approximately two years, this was my basic diet:

I. On Waking

One glass of warm water with half a lemon juiced into it. There are some health benefits to this. There is an article on the *Tasty Yummies* (n.d.)[31] website that lists 10 benefits of starting your day with this.

This would be followed by two more glasses of water, one with 1000mg of vitamin C and magnesium powder added.

II. Breakfast

I would eat at around ten thirty, after my morning exercise, daily quiet time (a time of reflection, reading my bible and prayer) and some admin work. These short periods (15 hours since supper of the previous evening) of intermittent fasting have certain long-term health benefits. Dr Mercola (n.d.)[32] sums this up in his article *Everything You Need to Know about Intermittent Fasting*:

- Fasting helps promote insulin sensitivity; optimal insulin sensitivity is crucial for your health, as insulin resistance or poor insulin sensitivity contributes to nearly all chronic diseases.
- It normalizes ghrelin (known as the hunger hormone) levels.
- It increases the rate of HGH production, which

has an important role in health, fitness and slowing the aging process.
- Fasting lowers triglyceride levels.
- Fasting helps suppress inflammation and fights free radical damage.
- In addition, exercising in a fasted state can help counteract muscle aging and wasting, and can boost fat-burning.

Breakfast consisted of:
- Three to four servings of fruit.
- I topped the fruit with a mix of 2-3 tablespoons of ground seeds and nuts which included flax seeds, almonds, pumpkin, sesame and sunflower. (Alternatively, I would soak the seed mix overnight and make a smoothie with the fruit and rice milk in the morning).
- Two to three apricot kernels (for the amygdaline).
- A cup of herbal tea (I enjoy drinking a variety of herbal teas, such as Rooibos, Honeybush, Green tea, Lemongrass tea, Rosehip tea, Lemon Verbena tea and Chamomile tea).

The fruit I consumed was predominantly seasonal, organic and where possible, sourced locally to ensure freshness. Below are some of the fruits available in the area where I live. You would need to source the seasonal fruits in your area.

Winter fruits: pineapple (contains digestive enzyme bromelain), papaya (contains digestive enzyme papain), various berries, bananas, guavas and citrus fruits.

Summer fruits: watermelon, melon, peaches, apricots, figs, prunes, grapes, pomegranates and plums.

III. Lunch:

My plate would be divided into 3 parts:
- ⅓ vegetable protein and starch
- ⅓ steamed vegetables
- ⅓ raw salad

I would add one or 2 of the below depending on my appetite:
- Ultra-InflamX (by Metagenics) drink or
- a cup of green or herbal tea, or
- freshly made vegetable juice.

Vegetables consist of: steamed broccoli, cauliflower, spinach, cabbage, asparagus, beans and carrots (at least two vegetables at a sitting).

Starch and vegetable protein consist of :Boiled sweet potato or butternut, tofu or the previous night's leftovers.

Note that for variety, the steamed vegetables were sometimes replaced by stir-fried vegetables, onions, herbs, garlic and ginger, with two spoons of olive oil.

Salad ingredients would consist of:
- Variety of herbal and salad greens

- Homemade sprouts
- Tomatoes, carrots and red pepper
- Avocado
- Seeds, herbs, onion and garlic
- Salad dressing of cold-pressed olive oil and lemon juice, apple cider vinegar, or a good fermented soya sauce.

If I had to rush somewhere I would have rice cakes with avocado or soy miso, but I would not recommend that now because of the high *glycemic index of rice cakes.

*The glycemic index is a value assigned to foods based on how slowly or how quickly those foods cause an increases in blood glucose levels.

IV.   Mid-afternoon Snacks:
- Two glasses of freshly-made vegetable juice.
- Soaked nuts: almonds, brazil nuts, pecans and walnuts.
- Dried fruit such as dates, prunes, figs and apricots (preferably organic and sulphur free).

Soaking the nuts and dried fruit make them easier to digest.

The above snacks would be consumed randomly between meals if I felt hungry. I always ensured that I had these on hand, so I wouldn't grab "junk food" to snack on.

V. Supper:
My plate would again be divided into 3 parts:
- ⅓ vegetable protein and starch
- ⅓ steamed vegetables
- ⅓ raw salad

Vegetable protein consisted of:
- Cooked legumes
- Soy tofu (soya bean curd)
- Mushrooms
- Quinoa (good protein source for vegans)

Starch was one of the followings:
- Brown rice or brown basmati rice
- Potato
- Sweet potato - boiled or baked in the skin
- Butternut - boiled or baked in the skin

Steamed vegetables:
(Sometimes I just had one kind, but mostly ate 2-3 different kinds of vegetables):
- Mainly cruciferous: broccoli, cauliflower, spinach
- Asparagus, carrots, beans, courgettes and peas

Fresh raw salad:
This included similar ingredients to those mentioned in the lunch menu.

Soups and Stews:

I ate these fairly often; especially during colder weather. The main meal would consist of soups or stews for lunch and supper. Ingredients consisted of vegetables, onion, garlic, ginger, legumes, herbs, sea salt or Himalayan salt and spices like turmeric, coriander, cumin, cinnamon, red and black pepper, and paprika.

I always included a fresh green salad and enjoyed another glass of vegetable juice or herbal tea after my meal.

VI. Dessert:

Dessert would be four soaked prunes, a piece of homemade dark chocolate, or chopped almonds and honey. Prunes are very high in antioxidants and prevent constipation. (The darker-skinned fruits and vegetables have very high antioxidant values.)

Before bed I would retire with a cup of chamomile tea to ensure that I slept well.

H. Evolving My Anti-Cancer Maintenance Diet

With time, experience and improvements in my physical condition, my diet began to develop and evolve.

I felt that my period as a vegan had served its purpose, and I continued to gain knowledge by studying and reading about health, particularly regarding cancer.

I am so grateful for the many wonderful experts who shared their knowledge, amongst them Dr Joseph Mercola and the many integrative medical doctors and natural practitioners presented on the documentary series *The Truth about Cancer*, hosted by Ty Bollinger.

The changes were predominantly along the lines of adding variation, improving preparation, and changing emphasis. These changes represented an evolving, rather than a rejection of, the previously discussed anti-cancer diet.

There were, however, a few ingredients that had to be dropped as new information came to light, such as unfermented soy and rice cakes.

I.   Animal Protein

Even though I followed a vegan diet for almost two years, with my present knowledge, I would only recommend a vegan diet for a shorter period of 6-9 months at the commencement of your treatment (for reasons discussed under *Why I Chose a Vegan Diet*, in chapter seven).

Animal protein provides a high-quality combination of all nine essential amino acids, while proteins from plant origin fall short on one or more of these amino acids. Though, a combination of vegan foods, containing different amino acids, can create full proteins. However unless one is committed to veganism this can be cumbersome. A good book outlining these combinations is *Diet for a Small Planet*, by Frances Moore Lappe.

The iron in animal protein especially red meat is also more easily absorb than the iron in vegetables This will helped me to prevent anaemia.

But I want to include a caution here, to only eat organic or free-range, grass-fed animal protein, because of the routine use of antibiotics and hormones in feedlots. I would also recommend including only small portions of animal products (about the size of ½ a palm of your hand for meat), 3-4 times a week. Bone broth is an excellent option as an animal protein, because it is easily absorbed by the body.

II. Fermentation of Grains, Nuts, Seeds and Legumes

According to Jennifer McGruther (*The Nourished Kitchen*,n.d.),[33] sprouting mung beans increases the absorbable iron by over 70 percent, compared to the untreated bean. Sprouting and roasting oats before preparing a breakfast porridge has been shown to increase zinc absorption by 55 percent and iron by 47 percent.

She points out that grains, nuts, seeds and legumes are potent sources of anti-nutrients, which include phytate and enzyme inhibitors. Anti-nutrients cause reduced mineral absorption and digestive problems, such as bloating, gas and allergies. However, soaking, souring, or sprouting these foods make the nutrients in them more bio available for absorption by the digestive system.

Grains, nuts, seeds and legumes are the main protein sources in the diet of especially vegans. It is therefore important that optimal nutrition and absorption is ensured.

Sally Fallon wrote a wonderful manual, called *Nourishing Traditions*, on how to prepare your food (mainly by fermentation) to optimize digestion of the nutrients.

III.   Exclusion of Unfermented Soy

I used legumes (beans and lentils), seeds, nuts, quinoa, miso, soy tofu and soy protein isolate as my vegan protein supply.

But I have since come to understand the dangers of unfermented soy. I do not eat any unfermented soy products at present for the reasons outlined here:

Reasons for excluding unfermented soy from your diet is outlined in *10 Soy Dangers* (The Weston Price Foundation)[34]:

- High levels of phytic acid in soy reduce assimilation of calcium, magnesium, copper, iron and zinc. Phytic acid in soy is not neutralized by ordinary preparation methods such as soaking, sprouting, and long, slow cooking, but only with long fermentation.
- Trypsin inhibitors in soy interfere with protein digestion and may cause pancreatic disorders.
- Soy phytoestrogens disrupt endocrine function and have the potential to cause infertility and to promote breast cancer in adult women.
- Soy phytoestrogens are potent anti-thyroid agents that cause hypothyroidism and may cause thyroid cancer. In infants, consumption of soy formula has been linked to autoimmune thyroid disease.
- Vitamin B12 in soy is not absorbed and actually increases the body's requirement for B12.
- Soy foods increase the body's requirement for vitamin D. Toxic synthetic vitamin D2 is added to soy milk.
- Fragile proteins are over-denatured during high temperature processing to make soy protein isolate and textured vegetable protein.
- Processing of soy protein results in the formation of toxic lysinoalanine and highly carcinogenic nitrosamines.
- Free glutamic acid (MSG), a potent neurotoxin, is formed during soy food processing and additional amounts are added to many soy foods to mask soy's unpleasant taste.

- Soy foods contain high levels of aluminium, which is toxic to the nervous system and the kidneys.

IV. Inclusion of Bone Broth

Most people with cancer have a problem with their intestinal flora. Bone broth lines the intestines and encourages the growth of beneficial bacteria. It also assists in healing the intestinal lining, and it did so for me.

Jordan Ruben explains in his book, *The Maker's Diet*, how bone broth healed his intestinal lining and helped save his life after he had been suffering from a severe stomach disorder. This book is well worth reading. He now produces a delicious bone broth powder that I use in my green smoothies. This can be ordered online from Organixx.com.

The Organixx website gives a list of the positive aspects of utilising bone broth in a feature called *Bone Broth Benefits*.[35] (They very usefully include references to each point they make, for those wanting to research the topic in more depth). Here is the list from the website:

- **Gut Health:** One of the main compounds that can support gut health is a specific type of gelatine found in bone broth, called a hydrophilic colloid.
- **Immune Support:** Grandma was right. Hearty homemade chicken soup, using a whole

healthy chicken (bones and all, in other words, a bone broth), is considered medicine by many people for good reason.
- **Joint Issues:** One of the ingredients in bone broth is collagen. Collagen can be very helpful for supporting healthy joints.
- **Healthy Bones:** Bone broth is high in calcium and magnesium. The slow cooking releases these vital minerals in a highly digestible and bio-available manner for your body.
- **Toxin-Fighting Power:** When the digestive system leaks toxins into the bloodstream, tiny particles of food are leaked as well. The body sees these foods as additional toxins to fight. Bone broth is high in gelatine, and gelatine has been shown to block these particles from entering the bloodstream.

Bone broth also encourages the formation of collagen in the body. My skin texture has improved dramatically since I've introduced bone broth to my diet.

V.   Green Smoothies

Freshly made smoothies full of fruit, vegetables and superfoods, are full of goodness and high in nutrition. They make a great breakfast or snack, anytime of the day. I particularly like green smoothies, because they not only boost your health but also combine many cancer-fighting ingredients, in a delicious way.

Green smoothies consist of a liquid base of water, coconut water, coconut milk or almond milk, and green leafy vegetables (kale or spinach). Add some fruit to the smoothie for sweetness. I like to add extras, such as cocoa powder, coconut oil, kefir and bone broth powder, to increase the nutritional value even further.

Reasons to drink green smoothies: *(Raw Blend* website, n.d.)[36]

- Green smoothies are easy to digest. When blended well, most of the cells in the greens and fruits are ruptured, making the valuable nutrients easy for the body to assimilate. Green smoothies literally start to get absorbed in your mouth.
- They are a fast, delicious way to increase energy. The goodness in green smoothies quickly makes its way to your cells to nourish, hydrate and energize.
- Green smoothies, as opposed to juices, are a complete food because they still contain fibre.
- They contain a dense mix of vitamins, minerals and phytochemicals which help build the immune system.
- By drinking green smoothies, you increase your consumption of chlorophyll. A molecule of chlorophyll closely resembles a molecule of human blood.
- Many people do not consume enough greens. By drinking two or three cups of green

smoothies daily you will consume enough greens for the day to nourish your body, and all of the beneficial nutrients will be well assimilated.

It is best to make your smoothies with fresh ingredients at home, because most store-bought smoothies are full of sugar, colourants and preservatives that have been added to enhance taste and shelf life.

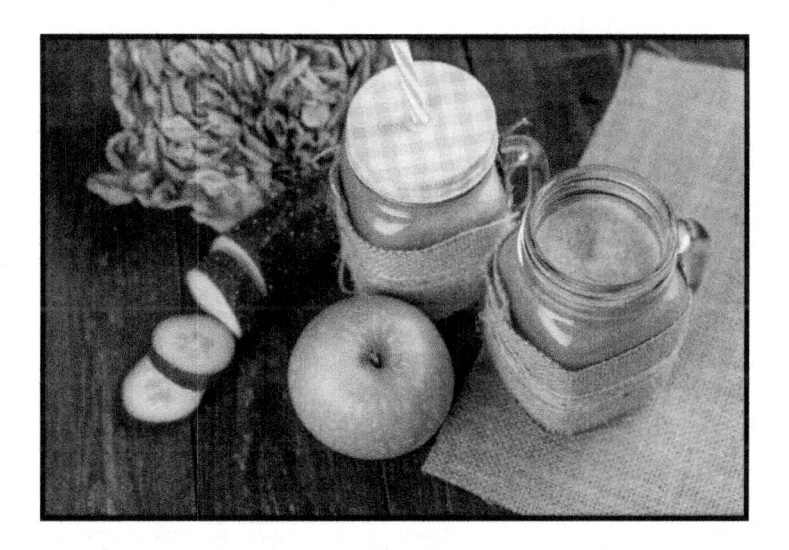

My Favourite Green Smoothie: (makes 1.7 litres)
2 bananas
1 cup of berries (strawberries, blackberries, blueberries, or any mix thereof) or
2 green apples
⅓ cup of pomegranate juice (freshly squeezed)

3 whole kale or spinach leaves
1 scoop of Organixx bone broth powder
½ cup soaked almonds
½ cup of kefir or coconut cream
½ lemon with a little rind still attached
2 tablespoons coconut oil
1 tablespoon cocoa
Filtered water to fill jug

Blend all ingredients together and enjoy!

VI.   Healthy Fats

Fats help us to absorb vitamins and offer many health benefits. Along with olive and avocado oil, I now also include coconut oil and organic butter from grass fed cows into my diet. Butter supplies omega 3 as well as vitamin D, but also contains many other benefits, besides being a delicious addition to the diet.

Below find some benefits of butter from Dr Axe. For those who want to delve a bit deeper, he includes studies and references in this article on his website. (n.d.)[37]

- **Anti-Inflammatory:** By consuming grass-fed butter, you directly increase your intake of butyric acid, which can decrease inflammation.
- **Better for Heart Health:** A heart study published in the journal Epidemiology looked at the effects of butter and margarine on cardiovascular disease. They found that margarine consumption increased the risk

of coronary heart disease occurrence, while butter intake was not at all associated with coronary heart disease occurrence.
- **Excellent Vitamin A Source:** Vitamin A is essential to proper endocrine system function.
- **Energy-Boosting and Appetite-Suppressing Medium-chain Triglycerides (MCTs):** The MCTs found in butter (and coconut oil) can be converted immediately into fuel for your body's muscles and organs.
- **High in anti-cancer CLA (Conjugated Linoleic Acid):** This is a compound that can potentially help provide protection against different types of cancer, and helps the body store muscle instead of fat.

A word of caution: if you are lactose intolerant you may have to avoid butter because it does contain traces of lactose.

If you cannot eat butter, or would like to supplement it with another good source of fat, then coconut oil is a great choice.

Below is a shortened list of Ten Medically Proven Coconut Oil Benefits by Dr Axe [38]:
- Proven natural treatment for Alzheimer's disease.
- Prevents heart disease and high blood pressure.
- Cures urinary tract infection (UTI) and kidney infection and protects the liver.

- Reduces inflammation and arthritis.
- Cancer prevention and treatment.
- Immune system boost (antibacterial, anti-fungal and anti-viral).
- Improves memory and brain function.
- Improves digestion, reduces stomach ulcers and ulcerative colitis.
- Helps with fighting candida and yeast infections.
- Assists with hormone balance.

VII.   Fermented Vegetables, Milk and Drinks

The fermentation of vegetables and milk offers a wide variety of probiotics and digestive enzymes. In her book, *Nourishing Traditions*, Sally Fallon explains how to make these products yourself, but they are generally also available in health-food stores.

Sauerkraut is essentially cabbage that has gone through careful fermentation. Kefir, yogurt and cottage cheese are all fermented milk products. Kombucha is a fermented tea, while apple cider vinegar is made from fermenting apples. I make sure that at least two of these are on my daily menu.

Always use organic products for the fermentation process if possible. (See also chapter 8 on the "Gut and Cancer", for further explanation on the importance of fermented foods in restoring gut bacteria.)

VIII. Ayurvedic Spices

Turmeric, ginger, cinnamon, curcumin, cayenne pepper and black pepper are all Ayurvedic spices that have many health benefits. Ayurvedic spices are powerful antioxidants and can assist us to heal and stay healthy. Turmeric is of special interest because it contains the component curcumin.

Studies have shown that curcumin modulates growth of tumor cells and selectively kills tumor cells, and not normal cells. Curcumin has been shown to inhibit the proliferation and survival of almost all types of tumour cells. (Ravindran, Prasad & Aggarwal, 2009)[39]

Tumeric has many other health benefits. It is anti-inflammatory, can alleviate depression, improve brain function and can assist in preventing cancer.
It is said that using black pepper with turmeric significantly enhances the anti-inflammatory aspects.

Turmeric can be used in many dishes, like stews, stir-fries and soups. It can also make a very satisfactory hot drink (which I love).

My Soothing Turmeric Drink Recipe:
1 teaspoon of turmeric
½ teaspoon ginger
¼ teaspoon of cinnamon
⅛ teaspoon of black pepper

1 tablespoon of coconut oil
3 tablespoons coconut cream or milk
Fill the cup with boiled water and enjoy.

I find this drink energises me, as well as enhancing my mood. It is a very satisfactory drink for a cold winter's evening and could assist in relieving cold and flu symptoms.

Please note: use only organic non-irradiated spices to experience the full benefit. Irradiation could destroy some of the health benefits of the spices

8. The Gut and Cancer.

The gut, also known as the gastrointestinal tract, is a long tube that starts at your mouth and ends at your anal passage.

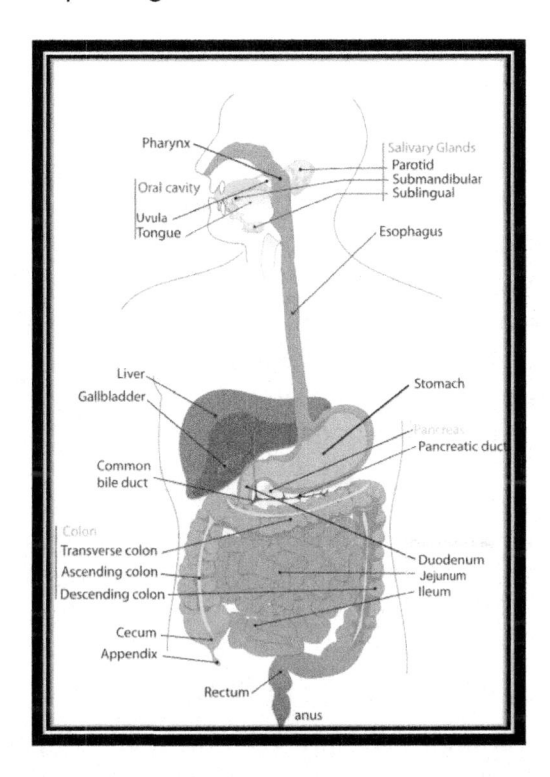

Its function, the processing and absorbing of food, and the excretion of wastes, is of vital importance for the functioning of the body. The gut houses the majority of our human bacteria: 10-100 trillion microbial cells, totalling on average around 1.6kg.

Two thirds of the gut microbiome (the population of bacteria in the intestine) is unique to each individual. Giulia Enders (as cited in Hopegood, 2015)[1], author of *Gut: The Inside Story Of Our Body's Most Underrated Organ*, says that "The gut is the largest sensory organ in the body, and has the second biggest collection of nerves, after the brain."

No wonder it is referred to as "the second brain" in alternative health circles. According to Dr Siri Carpenter (2012)[2]:

> Gut bacteria produce an array of neurochemicals that the brain uses for the regulation of physiological and mental processes, including memory, learning and mood. In fact, 95 per cent of the body's supply of serotonin is produced by gut bacteria.

Serotonin is a neurotransmitter and a natural mood stabiliser; the health of the gut affects the well-being of your body, mind and even emotions.

A. Cancer Gut Bacteria Connection.

The gut bacteria make up 70 per cent of your immune system. If they are thriving, they can launch successful attacks on invading, unhealthy, bad bacteria.

Wardill and Gibson (2017)[3] state:

The gut and immune system are closely linked. Just as our gut bacteria control our immune system, our immune system controls our gut bacteria. Research now suggests this interaction plays a significant role in determining cancer risk. Mice lacking certain immune molecules that slow the immune response, called anti-inflammatory cytokines, have more bad bacteria in their gut. This means a strong immune response ensures bad bacteria do not overpopulate our guts.

Most people with cancer have impaired digestive systems, damaged by years of abuse of refined carbohydrates, antibiotics, toxins, metals and especially stress.

My situation was no different. I suffered from bouts of constipation - a warning sign that my gut health was less than optimal. We are created to digest, assimilate and eliminate in perfect balance so that we can stay in good health.

According to Jennifer Brubaker (2017)[4]:
Women with breast cancer have an higher abundance of Enterobacteriaceae, staphylococcus and Bacillus when compared to women without breast cancer. Lactobacillus acidophilus, a familiar probiotic found in yogurt and kimchi, can reach the mammary gland and has a number of anti-cancer effects. Women who

ingest fermented milk products may experience protective antioxidant effects.

B. Foods to Restore the Gut.

You don't have to despair if your gut is less than optimal, as you can correct it. You can alter the composition of your gut flora positively by eating a variety of prebiotic and probiotic foods.

It is imperative to remove all processed foods, as well as foods which are high in sugar and chemical additives from your diet. They are a sure way to decimate the beneficial bacteria in your gut, allowing the harmful pathogenic type to thrive.

Prebiotic Foods.
Food that is prebiotic contains ingredients (mostly fibre) that gut bacteria feed on, producing fermentation by-products that benefit health.
Here are some of the most potent prebiotic foods:
- Almonds
- Asparagus
- Bananas
- Burdock root
- Cereal grains
- Chicory root
- Garlic
- Greens (especially dandelion greens)
- Mushrooms
- Oats
- Kiwi

- Leeks
- Legumes

Probiotic-rich Foods

Probiotic-rich foods are prepared by allowing bacteria to ferment food naturally. Common bacteria, like Lactobacilli, break down the sugars into acids, preserving the food and imparting a salty, tangy flavour.

Fermented foods can provide an instalment of healthy bacteria into the gut. The new bacteria enhance the diversity of our gut microbes to help the present bacteria do their job better.

Below are some of the most potent probiotic foods:
- Fermented vegetables (kimchi, sauerkraut, lacto-fermented pickles, traditional cured olives)
- Fermented soybeans (miso, natto, tempeh)
- Cultured dairy products (buttermilk, yogurt, kefir, cheese)
- Cultured non-dairy products (yogurt and kefir made from organic soy, coconut, etc.)
- Fermented grains and beans (lacto-fermented lentils, chickpea, miso, etc.)
- Fermented beverages (kefir and kombucha.)
- Fermented condiments (raw apple cider vinegar)

Repairing the gut can take some time, but by continuously eating foods which add good bacteria to your gut will correct it over time. Repairing the bacteria in the gut not only assist in the healing of cancer but can also ensure your general wellbeing and mood.

Dr Joseph Mercola (2012,2016)[5,6] on his website sets out the steps that can be taken to correct the gut bacteria. He gives a list of steps which should be followed and those which should be avoided.

His steps to correct your gut bacteria are:
- Eat plenty of fermented foods. Healthy choices include lassi, fermented grass-fed organic milk such as kefir, natto (fermented soy), and fermented vegetables.
- Take a probiotic supplement.
- Boost your soluble and insoluble fiber intake, focusing on vegetables, nuts, and seeds, including sprouted seeds.
- Get your hands dirty in the garden. Exposure to bacteria and viruses can serve as "natural vaccines" that strengthen your immune system and provide long-lasting immunity against disease.
- Open your windows. For the vast majority of human history, the outside was always part of the inside, and at no moment during our day were we ever really separated from nature.
- Wash your dishes by hand instead of in the dishwasher.

The following should be avoided:
- Antibiotics, unless absolutely necessary, and when you do, make sure to reseed your gut with fermented foods and/or a high quality probiotic supplement.
- Meat from animals raised in a Concentrated Animal Feeding Operation (CAFO), which are routinely fed low-dose antibiotics, as well as GMO grains loaded with glyphosate.
- Chlorinated and/or fluoridated water.
- Processed foods. Excessive sugars, along with otherwise "dead" nutrients, feed pathogenic bacteria.
- Agricultural chemicals, glyphosate (Roundup) in particular is a known antibiotic and will actively kill many of your beneficial gut microbes.
- Antibacterial soap, kill off both good and bad bacteria and contribute to the development of antibiotic resistance.

9. Parasites and Cancer

If having a parasite in your body is a scary thought for you, you're not alone. But parasites are far more prevalent than you think. The most common parasites found in the gut are roundworms, tapeworms, pinworms, whipworms, hookworms and helminths.

Because parasites come in so many different shapes and sizes, they can cause a myriad of symptoms, not all of which are related to digestion. But certain parasites can lead to cancer.

An article by the American Cancer Society (2016)[1] states:
> Certain parasitic worms that can live inside the human body can also raise the risk of developing some kinds of cancer. These organisms are not found in the United States, but they can be a concern for people who live in or travel to other parts of the world. Schistosoma haematobium is a parasite found in the water of some countries in the Middle East, Africa, and Asia. Infection with this parasite has been linked to bladder cancer. Possible links to other types of cancer are now being studied as well.

Dr Herman Spies diagnosed Schistosoma haematobium (the bilharzia parasite) as residing in me during our first consultation. He stated that the presence of these parasites was one of the main contributing factors towards the breast cancer.

According to Jens Rupp (2004)[2]:
> Bilharzia is a human disease caused by parasitic worms called Schistosomes. Over one billion humans are at risk worldwide and approximately 300 million are infected. Bilharzia is common in the tropics where ponds, streams and irrigation canals harbor bilharzia - transmitting snails. Parasite larvae develop in snails from which they infect humans, their definitive host, in which they mature and reproduce.
>
> Adult Schistosome worms are about 1 cm long and hang out in mesenteric veins (the small veins that carry blood from the intestine to the liver). The worms feed on red blood cells and dissolved nutrients such as sugars and amino acids. This can cause anemia and decreased resistance to other diseases. Schistosomes live in pairs, the male holding and protecting the female inside his ventral groove. Once paired, the two remain in constant copulation. The female lays hundreds of eggs each day, which find their way out of the human body through the urine or the faeces, depending on the species.
>
> The pathology is mostly caused by the large number of eggs becoming stuck in various body parts, in particular the liver (causing liver enlargement and malfunction) and the kidneys

(causing kidney damage, detectable by blood in the urine).

I started to experience anaemia in my late twenties and the doctors couldn't diagnose the cause. The problem was temporarily "fixed" with iron supplementation, but the cause remained.

10 Signs You May Have a Parasite:

Dr Amy Myers (2013)[3] lists these telltale signs of parasites in your body.
- You have unexplained constipation, diarrhoea, gas, or other symptoms of irritable bowel syndrome (IBS).
- You travelled internationally and remember getting traveller's diarrhoea while abroad.
- You have a history of food poisoning and your digestion has not been the same since.
- You have trouble falling asleep, or you wake up multiple times during the night.
- You get skin irritations or unexplained rashes, hives, rosacea or eczema.
- You grind your teeth in your sleep.
- You have pain or aching in your muscles or joints.
- You experience fatigue, exhaustion, depression, or frequent feelings of apathy.
- You never feel satisfied or full after your meals.
- You've been diagnosed with iron-deficiency anaemia.

Once a person is infected with a parasite, it's very easy to pass it along. If you have a parasite and don't wash your hands after using the restroom, you can easily pass microscopic parasite eggs onto anything you touch. It's also very easy to contract a parasite when handling animals.

Hand washing is an important procedure in preventing parasite contamination and transmission.

Travelling overseas is another way that foreign parasites can be introduced to your system. If you consume any contaminated water during your travels, you may acquire a parasite of some kind.

How to Deal with Parasites

My friend Suret Morkel (from Innerfruits.com) recommends a cleanse every six months, using Micro Sweep. It contains taheebo, grapefruit extract, wormwood, echinacea, olive leaf extract and clove. I use this product to assist in detoxification of fungal yeast and parasites.

In addition to the herbal remedies I also used the Rife machine, utilising the program designed to kill parasites (see the section on the Rife machine in chapter five), as well as the Parasit electromagnetic drops made by Dr Spies, which are specifically formatted to kill parasites in the body.

Dr Hulda Clark is an expert on cleaning out parasites. It is worth visiting her website (Clark, 2018).[4] Though many herbs have anti-parasitic properties, Dr Clark discovered that three herbs alone can rid you of over 100 types of parasites. These herbs are black walnut hulls, wormwood and common cloves. For the complete chart listing her recommended parasite cleanse see Addendum A at the back of the book.

10. Coffee Enemas for Detoxification

Breast Cancer was a sure sign to me that there was a toxin build up in my body. I needed to do as much as possible to clear it. I've already mentioned that I suffered from constipation, bloating and gas. It was therefore imperative to get the colon and liver cleared from toxins to work optimally again. Because of the well-documented benefits of coffee enemas in the treatment of cancer, I used them as a method to clear out toxins and ultimately heal the cancer.

Angela Doss (as cited in Wilson, 2018)[1] says the following:

> A 1982 study by the National Research Council (NRC) in the United States showed that coffee enemas have the power to reduce systemic toxicity by up to 700 percent. This is because caffeine and other beneficial compounds found in coffee -- when not consumed by mouth and therefore diluted by the digestive tract -- work together to stimulate the liver directly to increase production of glutathione S-transferase (GST). This is a powerful detoxifying enzyme that binds with, and flushes out, toxins in the body.

A. History of the Coffee Enema

An article in Wikipedia (1994)[2] states the following:

In 1920, German scientists investigated caffeine's effect on the bile duct and small intestines. Max Gerson proposed that coffee enemas had a positive effect on the gastro-intestinal tract. He claimed that unlike saline enemas, the caffeine travelled through the smooth muscle of the small intestine, and into the liver. This, he said, cleared even more of the gastro-intestinal tract and removed more toxins and bile than a normal enema. He told his patients often that the "coffee enemas are not given only for the function of the intestines but for the stimulation of the liver."

Coffee enemas are the primary method of detoxification of the tissues and blood in the Gerson Therapy. Cancer patients on the Gerson Therapy may take up to five coffee enemas per day. An article by The Gerson Institute (2017)[3] states the following:

> The purpose of the enemas is to remove toxins accumulated in the liver and to remove free radicals from the bloodstream....The purpose of the coffee enema is not to clear out the intestines, but the quart of water in the enema stimulates peristalsis in the gut. A portion of the water also dilutes the bile and increases the bile flow, thereby flushing toxic bile (loaded with toxins by the glutathione S-transferase enzyme system) out of the intestines.... A patient coping with a chronic degenerative disease or an acute illness can achieve the following benefits from

the lowering of blood serum toxin levels achieved by regular administration of coffee enemas:
- increased cell energy production
- enhanced tissue health
- better immunity and tissue repair and
- cellular regeneration
- relieve pain, nausea, general nervous tension and depression.

Even if you're sensitive to caffeine, taking coffee this way won't affect you. Don't use decaffeinated coffee though; you won't get the benefits.

Drinking coffee does not have the same benefits as the coffee enema. When drunk, the coffee passes through the digestive system and the stomach acids nullify the benefits that can be achieved from the enema.

B. Making and Using a Coffee Enema

This is the method and recipe I used for my coffee enemas. This recipe makes 6 cups of coffee. You will need:
- A stainless-steel pot
- 3 heaped tablespoons of ground organic coffee (fully caffeinated)
- 1.5 litre of filtered water
- Enema bucket

Recipe and method:

- Boil 1.5 litre of water in the pot and add 3 heaped tablespoons of coffee.
- Boil a further five minutes on low heat, then leave the coffee to cool down to room temperature. The coffee should rather be too cold than too warm.
- Pour the coffee into the enema bucket, using a sieve to prevent coffee grounds getting into the bucket.
- Rest the bucket on a shelf, about a meter from the ground.
- Use lubrication on the catheter to ensure ease of insertion.
- Lie down on the floor on your right side and insert the catheter.
- Open the clamp of the catheter and let two cups of coffee flow into the colon.
- Hold for at least 12 minutes. If you can't hold it for that long, allow the bowel to clean out.
- Continue by allowing another two cups of the remaining coffee to flow into the colon. Hold for 12 minutes.
- Continue by allowing another two cups of the remaining coffee to flow into the colon. Hold for 12 minutes.
- When finished rinse the bucket with boiling water and an antimicrobial agent.

The goal is to have two enemas that you are able to hold for 12 minutes each.

Do not do more than one enema per day for any extended period without medical supervision.

Always discontinue the enemas if there is any adverse reaction whatsoever, and discuss it with the doctor at your next appointment.

11. Lymphatic System and Drainage Methods

The infiltrating ductal carcinoma in my breast metastasized to a lymph node under my arm. This was classified as a metastatic ductal carcinoma.

Furthermore, the Quantec® healing sheets from Dr Spies also indicated other carcinoma in situ and other lumps in my body. It was clear that my lymphatic drainage was impaired and needed attention, to assist in healing the cancer.

To assist with understanding of the importance of the Lymph system and its function, below is a brief description of the system and its function taken from *quizlet.com*[1]

- The lymphatic system is a network of tissues and organs that lie just beneath the skin.
- The primary function of the lymphatic system is to transport lymph (a fluid containing infection-fighting white blood cells) throughout the body.
- The lymphatic system absorbs fats and fat-soluble vitamins from the digestive system and delivers these nutrients to the cells of the body, where they are used by the cells.
- It aids the immune system in removing and destroying waste, debris, dead blood cells, pathogens, toxins and cancer cells.

- The lymphatic system also removes excess fluid and waste products from the interstitial spaces between the cells.
- The lymph is moved through the body in its own vessels, making a one-way journey from the interstitial spaces to the subclavian veins at the base of the neck.
- The lumps that manifest in a human body are generally lymph nodes that are blocked.

My friend Elizabeth always refers to the body as a river, where the water needs to be flowing to ensure health.

I needed to enhance the way my lymph was flowing to regain my health and prevent any further blockages (lumps) from forming in the future.

There are hundreds of lymph nodes in the human body, as illustrated in the picture below. They are located close to the surface, such as under the arm, neck and groin, and also deep inside the body, such as around the lungs and heart.

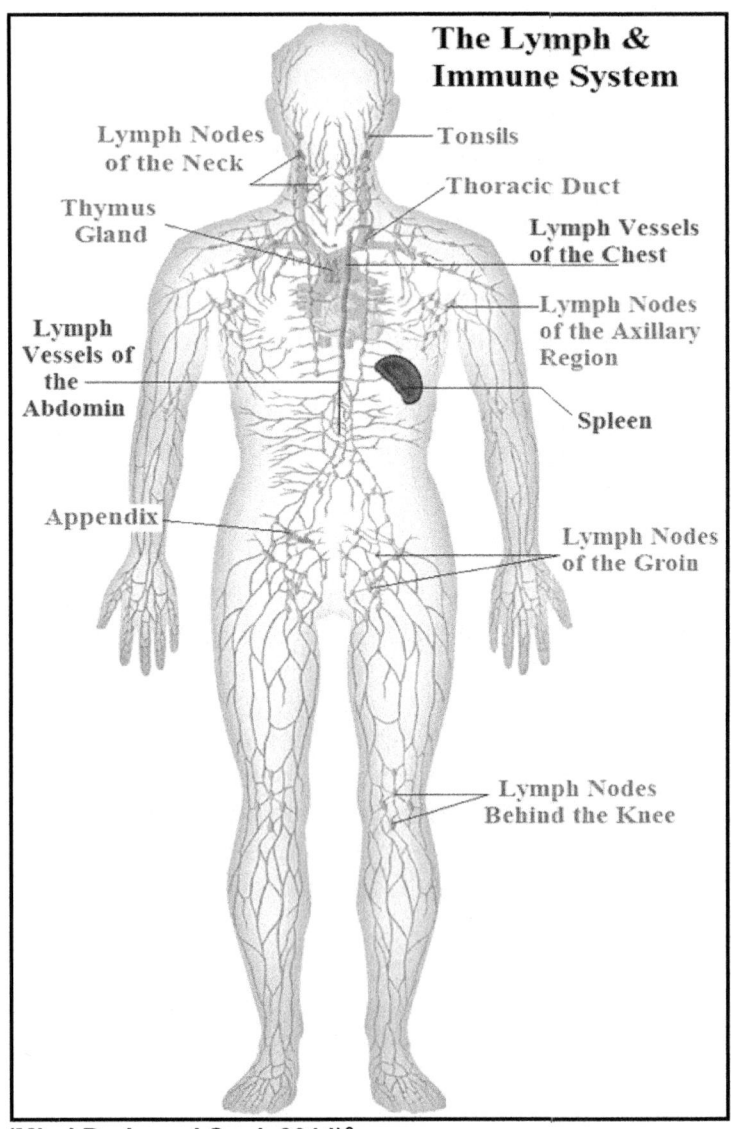

(Mind Body and Soul, 2014)[2]

Draining the lymph is vitally important. Below I have listed all the methods I used to drain the lymph in my body.

A. Gentle Lymph Self-Massage

We all love a good massage, but a lymphatic massage is a form of massage that specifically targets the flow of lymph in the body. It uses pressure and rhythmic circular movements to stimulate the lymph, encouraging its movement towards the heart for the drainage of fluid and waste.

Lymphatic massage has been shown in studies to push up to 78 per cent of stagnant lymph back into circulation. This mobilizes toxins for clearance, lessening the burden on the lymphatic system. ("Protocol-ID | TrulyHeal", 2018)[3]

Because of the swollen lymph nodes under my left arm and in my groins, I consulted with a lymph massage therapist who taught me how to gently massage the lymph to get it moving.

How to do a Lymph Self-Massage
You start massaging the lymph glands, using both hands and lightly performing 30-50 gentle, slow, pumping movements along the various nodes of the body. This is to move the lymphatic fluid that is just beneath the skin.
- Start at the base of the neck (the indentation above the collar bone) using your finger tips.

These are the Venus points (the drainage points for the head and the neck). Pump about 30-50 times.
- Then move to the side of the neck with downward pressure towards the Venus points.
- Follow by pulling the back of the neck towards the Venus points.
- Next move to under the armpits, another drainage point for the arms, chest and torso. Pump lightly 30-50 times.
- Stroke the top of the chest towards the armpits 30-50 times.
- Next, make gentle, upward strokes on the sides of the torso towards the armpit, using your hand.
- Lastly, make a big circular movement, using both hands, covering the groin and pubic bone all the way up to the rib cage and back, 30-50 times.
- Move back to the armpit and pump 30-50 times.
- In addition, the arms can also be gently pumped upwards to the armpits. The legs can be pumped towards the groin as well.

I continue to do the lymph massage every morning on waking up. The beauty of it is, it doesn't take much time and it makes you feel good and full of energy. At the same time, you are assisting lymph drainage and in doing so enhancing your health,.

Lymph massages are demonstrated beautifully by a massage therapist in a YouTube video series called Massage by Heather. (Wibbels, 2012)[4]

B. Lymph Pressure Massage or Air Therapy

Air Therapy consists of a set of body gloves into which you insert your legs, torso and arms. It is programmed for an alternating rhythm of inflation and deflation.

Pressure is applied, by the inflating cycle, to the parts of the body covered by the gloves, at a level that is completely comfortable. The application of pressure, to the tissue beneath the skin, moves from the end points of the limbs upwards towards the body's drainage points.

This treatment does the following to the lymphatic system (according to Dr Spies' website)[5]:
- It compresses the muscles, to aid in the removal of excess fluid from the tissues (as in a massage treatment).
- It is a non-invasive treatment, and the sensation is similar to a relaxing massage.
- The squeezing of the tissues and veins helps reduce pressure in the veins.
- It helps to oxygenate the tissues, thereby reducing the symptoms associated with lymph oedema and poor circulation.

I did 10 sessions of lymph pressure (Air Therapy) massages, recommended by Dr Spies, at his rooms. I enjoyed these sessions thoroughly and found it so relaxing that I fell asleep during many of the treatments.

C. Rebounding on a Small Trampoline

I discovered rebounding after my intense treatment period with Dr Spies.

Rebounding is one of the easiest ways to pump the lymph. It is the practice of jumping on a rebounder (a small trampoline) for 5-15 minutes. This passively moves the lymph while stimulating the circulation of blood throughout the body. Numerous studies have proven its efficacy, and an added benefit is that it also improves muscle tone.

It is more affordable to buy a rebounder than having to pay for regular massages. Besides, you can jump on the rebounder daily whenever it suits you. I bought a rebounder at a big department store called Game, which is similar to a Wal-Mart store in the USA, for R350. That is the price of one massage session by a therapist here in South Africa. Nine years later it is still in a good enough condition to jump on.

I rebound during the advertisements when watching my favourite soapie on television. An added benefit to having your own rebounder is that you can help your children or grandchildren to be more active as well. I find that most children love to jump on the rebounder when they come to visit.

D. Water

Lymph is about 95 per cent water, making water essential for its health. Stay hydrated by drinking around two litres (about eight glasses) of water a day. Without adequate water, lymphatic fluid cannot flow properly. One of the most common causes of lymph congestion is dehydration.

You can improve the lymph drainage process by adding lemon to your water. Lemon is an alkaline fruit that helps to mineralize the body and lymph. I start each day with half a lemon in a glass of warm water. Besides helping the lymph, it also helps the liver and gall to detoxify. I drink another glass of water with minerals added (including vitamin C) directly after this.

Ensure that you drink pure water by using a set of under-basin filters through which your tap water passes. Even better is pure spring water. Just be aware that reverse osmosis filters take minerals out of the water and waste a lot of water as well.

It is also a good idea to use a filter for your shower. Our skins absorb the chlorine and other toxins in normal unfiltered tap water, especially during a hot shower in which your pores open up.

E. Castor Oil Packs

Castor oil packs have been said to help improve liver detoxification, improve lymphatic circulation and reduce inflammation. I used them every 3-5 days over a period of a year. Below is how to do the castor oil packs:
- Use a piece of cloth about 4cm by 2.5cm and moisten it with castor oil.
- Place it over the stomach or the area that you want to treat - directly on the skin for at least an hour.
- Cover the cloth with a plastic sheet.
- Place a heat source on top of it. (I use a heated bean bag.)
- Cover yourself with an old towel or blanket to keep warm.
- I find it very comforting to lie down for the hour and listen to some good healing music.

The most common organs that castor oil packs are used for are the liver, gallbladder and the intestines.

There are detailed instructions on making and using castor oil packs at the *Wellness Mamma* website. (Katie-Wellness Mamma, 2018)[6]

The castor oil pack came to my rescue when I experienced pain in the gallbladder area (located on the right side of the body, just under the rib cage). I faithfully applied the patch an hour a day for a week.

Amazingly, the pain disappeared completely after that week. I concluded that it was most likely the gallbladder duct that was blocked, and it was opened up through this treatment.

F. Infrared and Ozone Saunas

There are many benefits to an infrared sauna session:
- It detoxifies heavy metals and removes BPA Bisphenol A (BPA) - a synthetic compound found in plastics) from the body. You can read more about BPA in a study published in the *Journal of Environmental and Public Health*, (2011).[7]
- The far infrared light penetrates the skin deeply and helps to detoxify impurities from the skin and lymph.
- An infrared sauna session enhances endurance and muscular performance.
- It helps with weight loss, not only due to calories burned (perhaps up to 800 calories per 30 minutes), but also because of the toxins removed from your body and fat cells.
- The fact that it detoxifies your body of heavy metals, might assist the immune system to ward off and fight cancer.

Don't forget that an infrared sauna will make you sweat a lot of water (and toxins), so you need to replace the lost electrolytes and minerals (such as potassium and magnesium).

To do this take a teaspoon of Himalayan sea salt (which contains over 80 trace minerals). A dose of magnesium and potassium at night before bed will help to prevent symptoms like muscle cramps and spasms.

Ozone Saunas are great to assist the lymphatic system to detoxify and function better.
Ozone saunas assist the functioning of the lymphatic system through the provision firstly of heat, which opens the pores in the skin, and then by introducing ozone. Ozone is a molecule containing three oxygen atoms. (The chemical symbol is O3.)

The ozone sauna works because the extra oxygen atom splits off fairly easily, resulting in a single O (oxygen) atom and an O2 (oxygen) molecule. The O atom can attach to pollutants and assist in moving them out, while the O2 that remains oxygenates the body. (*Oxygen Healing Therapies* website, 2017)[8]

The benefits of an Ozone Sauna are as follows:
- It detoxifies the body. It oxidizes toxins, so that they can be eliminated through the skin, lungs, kidneys and colon.
- It stimulates the immune system. It also stimulates vasodilatation of peripheral blood

vessels, assisting in relieving pain and speeding up the healing process.
- The sauna purifies the blood and lymph system by eliminating all kinds of bacterial and viral infections.
- It relaxes and loosens muscles by reducing the build up of lactic acid and helping injured muscles to repair more quickly.
- It reduce the chances that cancer will develop and spread.
- It boosts blood circulation.

G. Exercise

Movement not only combats adverse health conditions and disease, and stimulates the lymph, but is also good to uplift one's state of mind.

I walked for 30 minutes at least three times a week. I am fortunate to live in an residential complex with paths that run between bushes and plants, with views of the sea and the iconic and famous Table Mountain. I love walking on the beach as well, when the weather permits.

While healing from the breast cancer I also exercised in a ladies gym for 30-40 minutes, 2-3 times a week.

I enjoy exercising early in the morning, because I always feel great afterwards. Did you know that you release more than 20 endorphins during exercise?

University of Bristol researchers (as cited in *MailOnline*, 2008)[9] found that:
> Employees who enjoyed a workout before going to work-or who exercised during lunch-breaks were better equipped to handle whatever the day threw at them. It also found that people's general mood improved on days of exercise, but they became less calm on non-exercise days.

The research, published in *The International Journal of Workplace Health Management*, is the first of its kind to prove that exercise during work hours has mental, as well as physical benefits.

Here is a shortened list of some of the benefits of exercise, published by The Mayo Clinic (Mayo Clinic Staff, 2016, October 13)[10]:

- **Exercise controls weight:** Exercise can help prevent excess weight gain or help maintain weight loss. To reap the benefits of exercise, just get more active throughout your day - take the stairs instead of the elevator or rev up your household chores. Consistency is key.
- **Exercise combats health conditions and diseases:** Regular exercise helps prevent or manage a wide range of health problems and concerns, including stroke, metabolic syndrome, type 2 diabetes, depression, a number of types of cancer, arthritis and falls.

- **Exercise improves mood:** Physical activity stimulates various brain chemicals that may leave you feeling happier and more relaxed.
- **Exercise boosts energy:** Exercise delivers oxygen and nutrients to your tissues and helps your cardiovascular system work more efficiently. And when your heart and lung health improve, you have more energy to tackle daily chores.
- **Exercise promotes better sleep:** Regular physical activity can help you fall asleep faster and deepen your sleep. Just don't exercise too close to bedtime, or you may be too energized to hit the hay.
- **Exercise can be fun ... and social:** It gives you a chance to unwind, enjoy the outdoors or simply engage in activities that make you happy. Physical activity can also help you connect with family or friends in a fun social setting.

Exercise doesn't need to happen just in one workout session a day. You can get the benefit of exercise by doing various physical activities during the day, like taking the stairs instead of the lift, walking the dog, parking your car further away when going to the shops and walking the extra distance, or doing some stretching exercises when taking a break from your computer.

Aim for at least 30 minutes of exercise every day.

Also remember to check with your health practitioner before starting a new exercise program.

12. Thyroid and Iodine Connection

Dr David Brownstein's book, *Iodine: Why You Need It, Why You Can't Live Without It* (2009),[1] gave me knowledge of yet another piece of the puzzle of why I developed breast cancer.

Two years prior to the discovery of the lump in my breast I was feeling very tired. Initially I thought it was just the stress of moving to a new house in a different part of the city, but after a year my condition was still the same. I then suspected that this could be caused by my hormones that needed balancing and/or an underactive thyroid.

I went to see a medical doctor who was having success in treating patients with bio identical hormones. He started by carrying out various blood tests, which showed that my adrenals were exhausted. He also found that my thyroid reading (though still within the parameters of the medical chart readings) was on the low side. The doctor prescribed bioidentical hormones for the thyroid as well as for the adrenals.

I started to feel better almost immediately. But what I didn't know at that stage (as Dr David Brownstein explains in his book) is that you should always supplement with iodine when you take thyroid medication. Ideally, the iodine deficiency needs to be corrected before the thyroid hormone is given. The reason for this is that with the thyroid medication, the body's metabolic rate increases and therefore also the need for iodine.

In other words, if the thyroid hormone is given, while there is a deficiency of iodine, it will increase the body's need for iodine.

Dr Brownstein (2009)[2] explains further that:
> The thyroid gland and the breast have an advanced system for absorbing and storing iodine. When there is iodine deficiency, the breast and the thyroid glands enlarge to compensate for the deficiency. The iodine deficiency induces hyperplasia, which is a precancerous lesion. This sets the stage for a disease like breast cancer.

I would highly recommend Dr Brownstein's book. He writes about countless case studies from patients that he treated successfully over the years, using iodine combined with thyroid hormone.

I take small amounts of Lugol's Iodine Solution (two drops) together with a very low dose of thyroid medication daily to help my thyroid to function as normal. You can also get iodine from some foods, like seaweed and fish.

A. The Functions of Iodine in the Body.

Iodine is important to your thyroid for the production of thyroid hormones, but it also plays a role in the production of all the other hormones in the body. Even though a person only needs small amounts of iodine, it surprisingly also has antibacterial, anti-parasitic, antiviral and even anticancer properties. Adequate iodine levels ensure that the immune system functions properly.

According to Dr Brownstein, (2009)[3] "Every cell in your body contains and utilizes iodine. Iodine is concentrated in higher concentrations in the glandular system of the body. The thyroid gland contains a higher concentration of iodine than any other organ of the body."

A useful read about the functioning of the thyroid is found in the article *How does the thyroid work?* by *Pubmed Health*, (2015, January)[4]. The article explains that:

> The thyroid gland produces three hormones: triiodothyronine or T3, thyroxine or T4 and calcitonin. T3 and T4 increase the basal metabolic rate. They make all of the cells in the body work harder, so the cells need more energy too. This has the following effects, for example:
> - Body temperature rises
> - The heart beat becomes stronger and the pulse faster

- Food is used up more quickly because energy stored in the liver and muscles is broken down
- Brain maturation is promoted (in children)
- Growth is promoted (in children)
- Activation of the nervous system leads to higher levels of attention and quicker reflexes

Iodine plays a role during all phases of human development, even before birth. Expectant mothers should ensure that their thyroid levels are optimal to ensure normal growth of the foetus and prevent birth defects.

Normal functioning of the thyroid gland is vital for the growing child, in order to prevent mental development problems. Both children and adults need adequate iodine intake to prevent hypothyroidism and even hyperthyroidism. Iodine must be present in the diet or, if needs be, supplemented.

B. Iodine Deficiency and Breast Cancer

Aceves, Anguiano and Delgado (2005)[5] report that:
> Diets high in iodine are associated with low breast cancer rates. The authors suggest that iodine might prevent abnormal growth and division of breast cells, but further research is still needed to confirm this. A deficiency of iodine has been found to influence the

occurrence of many cancers, especially stomach and breast cancers. Many researchers have attributed the low rate of breast cancer in Japan to high dietary iodine (as well as selenium).

Elyn Jacobs (n.d.)[6] points out that:
Iodine is a critical mineral in the prevention of cancer and has been used in one form or another for centuries. It was used as medicine (for everything from breast cancer to syphilis) and consumed in the form of seaweed, and eventually added to the ingredients in bread. Then, in 1948, iodine was suddenly thought of as a dangerous substance and was removed from medical arsenals – as well as from food in the 1970s.

Jacobs also mentions a research paper which shows that iodine changes the gene expression of breast cancer cells. (You can read further about this in the article by Jacobs, listed in the references at the end of this chapter.)

Michael B. Schachter, MD, (2005)[7] states:
The commonly accepted medical opinion is that iodine's only role in the body is to help make thyroid hormones. Although this is an extremely important function, Abraham demonstrates that the role of iodine in the body goes far beyond its function of making thyroid hormones. Other possible functions include: helping to regulate moods, preventing cancer (especially in

breasts, ovaries, uterus, prostate and thyroid gland). He states, "All things considered, I think that the therapeutic use of iodine/iodide has the potential of drastically changing how medicine is practiced today".

A Special Note If You Are Considering a Therapeutic Iodine Protocol

It is always advisable to consult with a qualified health practitioner who can guide you on dosages suitable for your body, health condition and lifestyle.

According to David Brownstein, MD, and other iodine researchers, those on a high-dose iodine protocol (12.5 mg or 2 drops – 50 mg/day or 8 drops) may need a daily companion dose of magnesium as high as 1200 mg. Other companion nutrients are selenium, vitamin C, riboflavin, niacin and unrefined salt.

These nutrients will boost absorption and help prevent side effects from the protocol, such as headaches and fatigue.

13. Emotions and Stress

The brain controls all the signals that are sent to the body. It is important to understand the connection of our brain, thoughts and emotions to the resultant health or lack of health in the body.

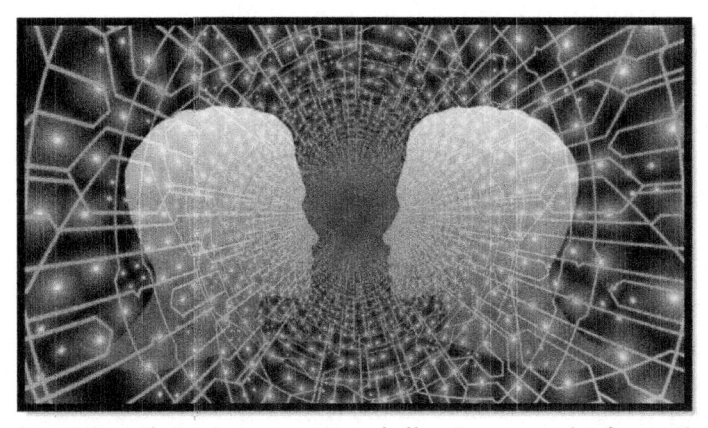

Emotional trauma, especially trauma before the age of four, has a huge influence on our emotional well-being. Even if you don't remember, the body does, and the body keeps the score. (The phrase "the body keeps the score" was coined by Bessel van der Kolk, M.D.)

Emotional trauma essentially gets placed into the unconscious part of our brain. It then becomes translated into the body and nervous system and can result in many health problems. One of the health issues is interference with sleep. Not being able to sleep affects the lymph drainage system, which in turn affects the detoxifying of the brain and body.

Fear, hate, shame and other negative emotions cause limiting beliefs and stress that play through into your thoughts. Your thoughts play back into your emotions. These emotional and thought patterns radiate out into every part of life.
The good news is that we have the ability to rewire the brain. It is possible to change the thoughts, habits, patterns and beliefs that keep us stuck in destructive behaviour that could later harm our health.

Dr Caroline Leaf, Ph.D., has been involved in medical research on the brain for over 25 years. She explains scientifically in her book, *Switch on Your Brain* (2013),[1] how thoughts affect brain function:
> If you are concentrating on thoughts of fear, anxiety, bitterness, self-hatred, rejection, guilt, condemnation, unforgiveness, anger, rage, resentment and so forth – your brain is full of toxic memories that will make you sick. Your hypothalamus is going to respond by producing insufficient or excessive quantities of certain chemicals which then become toxic and harmful for you and leads to the development of disease.

She found that scientists using brain imaging techniques were able to observe the difference in the images between someone who has had negative or 'unhealthy looking' thought patterns and then has changed these to positive or 'healthy looking' thought patterns. These thought patterns affect the matter in the brain and in turn affect every cell in your body, your emotions and ultimately, your health.

She promotes that you can retrain your brain and change these patterns. This will assist in the return of health to your body and mind. In this book Dr Leaf outlines a method she claims will enable a change in thinking patterns, or what she calls detoxification in the brain, in a 21 day period.

Candace Pert, Ph.D., neuroscientist and pharmacologist and one of the pioneers of psychoneuroimmunology, states in her book *Molecules of Emotion* (1997)[2] that the chemicals that are running our body and our brain are the same chemicals that are involved in emotions.

It is clear that we should be giving attention to detoxifying the brain and emotions to stay healthy.

This ought to be carried out every day, the same way you would eat vegetables to stay healthy for the rest of your life.

Healing Stress and the Emotions
The most powerful transformation in my life- physically, mentally and emotionally-involved a

radical change in mindset and a challenging of old belief systems.

Initially, I didn't think that my emotional state was a major contributor to the breast cancer. I didn't understand how negative emotions deplete your energy and strength and therefore your immune system. Sickness, especially cancer, thrives on a depleted immune system.

So how did I discover that emotional health is vital for healing cancer?

During my first appointment with Dr Herman Spies, he made me aware of the importance of healing my emotions. He explained that healing cancer is dependent on the physical, emotional and spiritual aspects of a person's life. He also emphasized that without emotional restoration, healing the cancer would be compromised.

As mentioned previously, I was presented with Quantec® healing sheets after every consultation. These listed all the physical and emotional issues identified, at cellular level, by the scan at that point in time.

While receiving the high-dose vitamin C intravenous drips (which normally took about an hour), I would read through the report. I started to identify some of the emotions to be true in my life, and became more interested in the emotional analysis and the applicable affirmations for healing. These were predominantly taken from Louise L. Hay's book, *You can Heal your Life* (2004)[3].

I've since bought myself this book and find chapter fifteen, *The Lists*, very helpful. This chapter deals with the physical problem, cause of the emotional reason for problem and the new thought pattern that needs to be adjusted to.

But it was only after I discovered *The Healing Codes Manual*, by Dr Alexander Loyd and Dr Ben Johnson (2004),[4] that I truly found an effective way to journey towards emotional and physical healing.

The Healing Codes, a self-healing method that helps you to remove stress (the primary cause of illness and disease) from your body, was discovered by Dr Alexander Loyd in 2001. Here is a extract from his book:

> Practicing "The Healing Codes" activates your body's natural healing centres in order to identify and heal negative cellular memories that shut down your immune system and keep you from optimal health. Using a combination of techniques like prayer, meditation and affirmations, "The Healing Codes" have helped thousands of people from all over the world correct physical, emotional, relational and success issues.

The Healing Codes states that it works on the following principles:
- Wrong beliefs are the cause of the majority of the problems in one's life.
- Wrong beliefs are destructive interpretations of internal images.
- Wrong beliefs motivate thoughts, feelings, and harmful actions that cause pain to ourselves and those around us.
- Wrong beliefs cause us to misinterpret our current circumstances as threatening. This causes our nervous system to go into a flight or fight mode, and therefore into permanent stress mode.
- It is this stress that has been found to cause 95% of all health problems.
- Stress also causes our cells to shift into self-protective mode.
- Stress in our nervous system will eventually lead to illness, pain and suffering.

I decided to commit myself to "Phase One: 12 Days to a Changed Life" in the *Healing Codes Manual*.

It was an eye opener to discover all the "wrong beliefs"- how they were affecting my stress levels and therefore my health, well-being and thinking, and how this resulted in my breast cancer.

I discovered, through *The Healing Codes*, that my main destructive emotion was fear. This caused a tremendous amount of insecurity and anxiety, which turned into stress. Instead of enjoying good times, I would be waiting for things to go wrong. I expected my present happiness to be derailed by difficulty, pain, sorrow, turmoil, and, loss of money and well-being.

According to a researcher at Stanford University, Bruce Lipton PhD and author of *The Biology of Belief* (2005),[5]

> Stress originates from wrong beliefs which cause us to misinterpret our circumstances as threatening, and ourselves as being threatened. This causes internal stress and sends the body and its cells into a "flight or fight mode" that can cause sickness and disease over time.

Just before the diagnosis of the breast cancer, certain emotional symptoms were increasing in magnitude and caused me to be in constant stress. Fear caused me to:
- Prepare myself for the worst
- Hold back love
- Be in turmoil
- Experience excessive frustration with difficult situations
- Think that others would take advantage of me
- Be unkind
- Not trust that things would work out for the good

- Have pride
- Try to control everyone and every situation

The Healing Codes guided me to discover the root of the wrong beliefs that caused the fear and anxiety in my life. To do this, it was important to identify the event that had led to the wrong beliefs. (This is normally an event that happens before the age of four.)

I discovered that the fear and insecurity that ruled my life, took root when I was only seven months old. My wonderful, caring mother had suddenly fallen very ill. She'd been diagnosed with tuberculosis and was forced to immediately stop breastfeeding me. She'd been hospitalised and left me in the care of my loving grandmother.

As I delved into the emotions around this, I became aware that it was this dramatic and sudden separation that caused me to expect things to go wrong in my life.

Once I discovered where my anxiety and fear originated, and the associated wrong beliefs connected to them, I could replace these with "truth statements". Only then could I truly start to experience joy and peace and all the other virtues that would assist me to live in the relaxed state of mind that would lead to health.

The 12-day program changed my life and my outlook. I started to experience the world differently. Life became easier, lighter, full of hope and purpose. I experienced more peace, more patience, more love and more joy, and less stress. It was easier to focus on the positive.

My own family and friends noticed the changes in me and even today my son and husband still remark sometimes on how I have changed since discovering *The Healing Codes*.

Besides all the positive emotional changes, my skin started to heal, and at present I can honestly say that I am truly comfortable in my skin. This after suffering from severe eczema for most of my life.

I use my skin as a barometer for my emotional state and stress levels. The appearance of eczema quickly indicates when some wrong belief, connected to negative emotions, needs to be replaced with "truth statements".

There are many other ways that you can lessen your stress and change your mood. Hiyaguha Cohen (March 2017),[6] at the *Baseline of Health Foundation* website, suggests some steps to take. Below is a shortened version of the list:
- Use Affirmations: The way we talk to ourselves greatly influences our outlook on life. By consciously changing negative messages to

positive messages, we can literally brainwash ourselves into a more upbeat frame of mind.
- Use Prayer: Praying takes the load off of ourselves and passes it on to a higher being who has the power to effect change for the better. An example of a short prayer: "God grant me the serenity to accept the things I cannot change, the courage to change the things I can, and the wisdom to know the difference."
- Exercise…tai chi, chi gung, yoga: Any kind of exercise can distract the mind from its obsessions.
- Keep a Gratitude Journal: Write down five to seven things for which you're grateful for that day. At the end of each week, review your journal, and you'll soon see that no matter how dismal your circumstances, you still have a number of things to cherish.
- Meditate: One of the best ways to take a break from the worries and negative thoughts assailing you is to simply stop thinking for a while. Meditation is like taking a short vacation from the mind's obsessions.
- Take a break from the news: The news can be depressing and can lead to plenty of doomsday-type thinking.
- De-Clutter: A cluttered life helps sustain a cluttered, unhappy mind. Make a list of the top 10 annoyances that you haven't had time to fix or deal with. Then, make a commitment to

tackle one annoyance each week until you've finished clearing up your entire list.
- Share feedback with your partner: Make it a daily ritual to spend 15 minutes with your partner offering and receiving appreciation, even if you're fighting. You can also use the time to talk about whatever feelings you're experiencing. Not only will you develop greater intimacy, but you'll also find that life seems a whole lot brighter.
- Surround yourself with positive images: Choose artwork that inspires you. If everywhere you look in your home and office ignites joy in you, it will be much easier to stay on the "sunny side."
- Listen to what you love. Music has enormous power to energize and uplift.

When I felt negative, tired or stressed I would listen to half an hour of calm relaxing music. Positive thoughts and increased energy levels would follow. I really enjoy two particular artists and their special compilations.

- The first is Jonathan Goldman and his *Holy Harmony* music.
- The second is Michael Tyrrell of Wholetones and his *Healing Frequencies Music Project*.

Today I understand how important it is to limit stress and negative emotions in my life, in order to ensure happiness and health.

14. The Importance of My Faith in God

I am a Christian and believe in God the Father, Jesus Christ, and, the Holy Spirit.

My faith in God has played a major role in my healing journey. It was the promises in the Bible that encouraged and strengthened me to follow the alternative path to healing. The Word of God, especially the Psalms, was a great comfort to me and assisted greatly in banishing fear from my mind and replacing it with trust.

I do believe God can perform miracles and heal instantaneously, but in my case, the instantaneous miracle didn't happen. However, this didn't stop me from believing that God would supply everything I needed for life and godliness, and that healing through a process would happen.

In the Bible, 2 Peter 1:3 states, "His divine power hath given unto us all things that pertain unto life and godliness, through the knowledge of Him that hath called us to glory and virtue." (21st Century King James Version, 1994).

I understood a little about the healing power of the body but didn't fully comprehend its God-created ability to heal itself. We just have to give it the right input - spiritually, emotionally and physically.

If we live according to the principles taught by Jesus, which are essentially the blueprints of the One who designed us and formulated the way we should live, then this should assist our bodies and minds to exist in a general state of health. Some of the spiritual principles to live by are - love, forgiveness, trust, joy, peace, patience, kindness, goodness, humility and self-control. We are to live without worry and fear, and the resultant peace should feed through into our bodies.

Love, one of the foundational principles, can be translated as respect, acceptance and appreciation for others, and for yourself, your body and the environment.

We're not to despair and become helpless in sickness. Illness is not God's punishment for sin. We can call out to God who is the giver of all good things, and who has promised ongoing forgiveness for anything we might have done to ourselves or others. I believed God heard my call to him for healing and supplied me with the wisdom to achieve it.

A. Discovering the Father's Love

This was one of the major spiritual insights that I was to acquire during my healing journey: God is

the FATHER of all and He LOVES everything He has made. Therefore He loves me.
I believed in God the saviour but didn't see and experience God as a father full of love, grace and compassion. Even though I confessed that God is love, somehow, I was still scared of a harsh God that could punish me for my wrongs.

It was important for me to understand that the breast cancer was not God's punishment. God's intention is always for us to be whole, healed and healthy. Jesus demonstrated this by showing compassion to all and healing all sicknesses he came across. He said, "if you have seen Me you have seen the Father." In other words, He came to show us what the Father's heart is towards us.

It is most often our own ways that cause us to get sick.

A friend lent me a book written by Joseph Prince (2007)[1], called *Destined to Reign: The Secret to Effortless Success, Wholeness and Victorious Living*. In this book Joseph explains God's love and good intention towards us. In it, he states the following:
> There is nothing you can do to make God love you more and there is nothing you can do to make him love you less. He loves you perfectly and he sees you clothed with Jesus' righteousness ....God blesses you not because you are good but because He is good.

The more strongly you believe this, and the more this truth gets a hold on the inside of you, the more it will change your thoughts and feelings, and the less you will fall victim to unhealthy emotions and behaviours.

God used this book to cement this truth deeply into my spirit, so I could see Him as 'Abba Father'. The word Abba was used by Jesus to address His Father and has within it the intimacy of the word we know as 'Daddy'.

Understanding the truth about God's love was very important for me, in terms of believing that I would be healed and not die.

The Bible is full of God's promises that confirm that if we ask, we will receive. One such promise is where Jesus said in Mark 11:24 (NIV Study Bible, 1985), "Therefore I tell you whatever you ask for in prayer believe that you have received it and it will be yours."

B. The story of King Hezekiah

The book of Kings, in the bible, contains an illustration of how we can ask God to lengthen our lives in 2 Kings 20:1-11. (NIV Study Bible, 1985). This passage of scripture describes how King Hezekiah fell very ill. The prophet Isaiah confirmed to Hezekiah that this was a sickness that was going to lead to death, and told him to put his affairs in order. Hezekiah then turned to the Lord and prayed to God to heal him. Hezekiah didn't feel he had fulfilled his purpose here on earth. He turned to God, and didn't doubt God's goodness and love.

The Lord heard Hezekiah's prayer and sends the prophet Isaiah back to him, to give him the following message, "Thus says the LORD, the God of your father David, 'I have heard your prayer, I have seen your tears; surely, I will heal you". He was then instructed to lay a cake of figs on his boils. Through this message of wisdom from God and the physical act of carrying it out, the Lord healed Hezekiah, and his life was extended by 15 years.

I identified with the story of Hezekiah because, like him, I basically had a disease that could lead to death. The doctor told me that if I refused radiation and chemotherapy, I would most likely not live another five years. Like Hezekiah, I also cried out to God to heal me and lengthen my life.

This piece of scripture encouraged me to believe that I would be healed too. It helped me to believe that God would keep me alive until I had fulfilled my purpose.

I was just 51 and felt that my purpose here on earth was not fulfilled, because I still wanted to be there as a mother for my son, Jonathan, who was 15 years old at the time.

Today, on reflection, I can say that I've seen Gods goodness and love. He healed me, not only from cancer, but also my emotions and thought life. I could see my son grow up and be there for him as a healthy mother.

In the bible, in Romans 8:28 (NIV Study Bible, 1985) it states, "And we know that in all things God works for the good of those who love him, who have been called according to his purpose." .

C. My Dream

Shortly after the diagnosis, I had a very vivid dream. I believe that God gave me the dream to assure me that I would be made whole, healed and healthy.

In the dream I was driving in a little car between vertical cliffs rising to the sky on both sides. These cliffs looked sharp, cold and dangerous, as if they could tumble down on me at any moment. I felt very scared and fearful.

After driving for a while, I started to see a bright, warm light far in the distance. As I eventually drove away from the cliffs, I was overwhelmed by the breath-taking beauty that appeared. I stopped the car, and as I got out I felt the warm sensation of the sun on my skin. The green grass felt soft under my feet as I made my way towards a waterfall cascading into a crystal-clear pool.

The sky was a bright blue, and the ground was covered in flowers with beautiful, vibrant colours. Different kinds of birds, also in bright colours, were singing joyfully. Trees in different shades of green were supplying fruit for birds and shade for others to rest under.

In my imagination, I perceive that paradise probably looks like this.

The dream was symbolic to me of my healing journey. The start of the journey was scary and frightening, but as I continued, I could see a light at the end of the tunnel as the faintest signs of my healing started appearing. The dream served as a promise to me that I would arrive at a stage in my life that represented health and vitality.

It was a confirmation that I would see the abundant goodness of the Lord in the years to come and that I would live and not die.

D. Spiritual Disciplines that Helped me on my Healing Journey

I. Prayer

After I shared with her my discovery of the lump in my breast, my friend Suret, suggested that I visit 'Healing Rooms' (a place the sick can go to be prayed for). Miraculously, a group had recently started a Healing Rooms ministry in my area. I saw this as God's provision.

The prayer sessions strengthened my faith. I always felt more positive, joyful and hopeful after being prayed for.

While praying for me at Healing Rooms, one lady had a vision of a bird that was joyfully singing from the heart. I interpreted this vision as a confirmation that I would be singing for joy over my healing. It also confirmed the dream I'd had, and strengthened my faith.

I prayed often on my own as well. During my prayer and meditation sessions, where I quieted my thoughts, God would give me insight into issues and emotions that needed dealing with in some way or another.

The Health Site (2015)[2] cites a study conducted by Lisa Miller, professor and director of Clinical Psychology and director of the Spirituality Mind Body Institute at Teachers College, Columbia University, concludes that there are benefits to prayer. Here are a few of the benefits she listed:
> Makes you stress free, reduces your chances of suffering from depression and anxiety, keeps away stress-related disorders, helps you deal with emotional onslaught, makes you happier and can speed up post-surgical recovery.

II. Counselling

The bible states in James 5:16 (Amplified Bible, 1987) "Therefore, confess your sins to one another (your false steps, your offenses) and pray for one another, that you may be healed and restored. The heartfelt and persistent prayer of a righteous man (believer) can accomplish much (when put into action and made effective by God—it is dynamic and can have tremendous power)."

The first thing I did after the diagnosis, was to find a godly counsellor. Pat was the person I chose, and she played a very important part in my healing.

I met Pat while attending a course on caring for the soul that she was running, nine years before my diagnosis. I recognized from the beginning that Pat loved the Lord deeply, and that she was a very wise practical person. Many people have benefited greatly from Pat's counselling, and I was one of them.

After Pat had agreed to counsel me, I met with her on a weekly basis for about six months. During these meetings tears were shed, and many prayers were prayed. Pat listened, counselled, read the Bible and prayed with me through many issues. She ministered to me with godly wisdom, prayer and deliverance.

As already mentioned in the previous chapter, negative, toxic emotions can assist in triggering the production of more cancer cells. It is therefore vitally important to confront deadly emotions like anger, bitterness, resentment, depression, unforgiveness and especially fear. A godly and experienced counsellor can be very helpful in leading you to recognise, admit and address toxic emotions. Forgiveness plays a major part in ridding oneself of destructive emotions.

Pat helped to build my faith and trust in God. The bible states in Hebrews 11:1 (Amplified Bible, 1987) "Faith is the assurance (confirmation, the title deed) or proof of things we do not see and the conviction of their reality to be (faith perceiving as real fact what is not yet revealed to the senses)."

She also helped me to overcome the fear of dying, so I could believe with all my heart and soul that I would be healed. The final overcoming and cutting loose from the fear of death happened seven months after the diagnosis, when I developed a sudden pain on my right side, below the waist.

The first thought that came to mind was that the cancer had now spread to other parts of my body. This was a fear planted by the surgeon after the diagnosis. She had told me that if I refused chemotherapy and radiation, that the cancer could spread throughout my body.

During our counselling session that week, Pat made me aware that no one can be sure of the future; all we can really be sure of is right now.

She said "One day at a time. Actually, one moment at a time."

I believe that God guided me to understand that the pain had something to do with a gallstone stuck in the bile duct. I treated myself by applying a hot castor oil patch every day for a week, and the pain went away, never to appear again.

A godly counsellor can also guide you in line with the wisdom of the Bible. For instance, with regard to anger, the Bible offers us the following advice in Ephesians 4:26, 31 & 32 (NIV Study Bible, 1985)

> In your anger do not sin: Do not let the sun go down while you are still angry....Get rid of all bitterness, rage and anger, brawling and slander, along with every form of malice. Be kind and compassionate to one another, forgiving each other, just as in Christ God forgave you.

I would highly recommend that you find yourself a counsellor, someone that you completely trust and can be 100 percent honest with.

III.   Reading Scripture
I meditated on the scriptures in the Bible daily.

The Psalms especially brought me great comfort and helped to build my faith. Many of the Psalms were written when David was distressed, and his life was in danger. David expresses his trust in God to protect him and bring him out of these circumstances.

The renewing of our minds happens as we read and meditate on scripture. I strongly believe that renewing the mind is very closely linked to having healthy emotions. The Bible tells us 365 times not to fear and it does this predominantly in relation to our irrational fears and anxiety. Fear is one of humanity's strongest emotions, and has been identified as the cause of many health problems which we experience. By believing that God loves you and that He has your best interests at heart, you can relax and let go of fear.

IV.   Singing

A new study by Tenovus Cancer Care and the Royal College of Music (2016)[3] has found that "Singing modulates mood, stress, cortisol, cytokine and neuropeptide activity in cancer patients and carers."

This study also found that cortisol levels were reduced after just one hour of singing in a choir. Singing therefore could reduce inflammation in the body, which is one of the causes of many diseases (including cancer).

I chose to participate in singing by worshipping God. The Bible encourages us, in many verses, to worship God. Singing is also an expression of thankfulness.

I visited churches where the worship was lengthy and of good quality. I also played worship CD's and sang along, especially after my quiet time (time spent reading the bible or meditating) in the morning.

V.   Speaking Words of Life.
I concentrated on speaking encouraging and positive words over myself and others. It is vitally important to speak encouraging, positive, and uplifting statements about yourself and others at all times. What you say today can become your reality tomorrow.

The Book of Proverbs (in the Bible) is a practical book of the sayings of King Solomon, who was known for his profound wisdom, and it gives useful guidelines for a good life. It has a lot to say about the words we speak. Here are a few examples:

"Death and life are in the power of the tongue, and those who love it will eat its fruit."(Proverbs 18:21, NASB, 1995)

"Your own soul is nourished when you are kind, it is destroyed when you are cruel."(Proverbs11:17, The Living Bible, 1971)

"A gentle answer turns away wrath but harsh words stirs up anger."(Proverbs 15:1,NIV Bible, 1987)

"The soothing tongue is a tree of life, but a perverse tongue crushes the spirit."(Proverbs 15:4,NIV Bible, 1987)

"Gracious words are a honeycomb, sweet to the soul and healing to the bones."(Proverbs 16:24,NIV Bible, 1973)

"The mouths of fools are their undoing and their lips are a snare to their very lives." (Proverbs 18:7,NIV Bible, 1973)

VI. Laughter

The Bible gives the following advice in Prov. 17:22 (Amplified Bible, 1987) "A cheerful heart is good medicine and a cheerful mind works healing, but a broken spirit dries up the bones (saps a person's strength)".

This scripture suggests that being cheerful and thus being prone to laugh, could assist in healing, and even keep you in good health.

Bellert (1989)[4] found that humour and laughter does improve one's mood and can form an adjunct therapy in oncology.

Dunbar (as cited in a New York Times article by Gorman, 2011)[5] says the following:

> Laughter is regularly promoted as a source of health and well being, but it has been hard to pin down exactly why laughing until it hurts feels so good. The answer, reports Robin Dunbar, an evolutionary psychologist at Oxford, is not the intellectual pleasure of cerebral humor, but the physical act of laughing. The simple muscular exertions involved in producing the familiar ha, ha, ha, he said, trigger an increase in endorphins, the brain chemicals known for their feel-good effect.

At the beginning of my healing journey, while driving to fetch my son at school, I stumbled upon a radio program on laughter. The guest speaker was talking about teaching people to laugh by starting with a fake laugh, which would then turn into real laughter. I initially thought that this was really silly, but once I started to practice it, I realised that it really works.

It seems that even if you fake laugh your body can still perceive it as real laughter.

I would practice laughter whenever I felt stressed, and noticed that my mood changed for the better after the laughing session. I would feel light, calm and joyful afterwards. As a family, we learned to use this principle of laughter to create joy and peace during stressful times.

Markham Heid (2014)[6], in an article on laughter and health benefits, refers to the work of Dr Lee Berk. An excerpt from the article states:

> Thanks largely to these stress-quashing powers, laughter has been linked to health benefits ranging from lower levels of inflammation to improved blood flow, Berk says. Some research from Western Kentucky University has also tied a good chuckle to greater numbers and activity of "killer cells," which your immune system deploys to attack disease. "Many of these same things also happen when you sleep right, eat right, and exercise," Berk says, which is why he lumps laughter in with more traditional healthy lifestyle activities.

Berk has even shown that laughter causes a change in the way your brain's many neurons communicate with one another. Specifically, laughter seems to induce "gamma" frequencies—the type of brain waves observed among experienced meditators. These gamma waves improve the "synchronization" of your neuronal activity, which bolsters recall and memory.

I tried to watch as many comedies as possible and read humorous books, that would encourage me to laugh out loud. I read many of Barbara Johnson's wonderful and funny books and these assisted me in my quest to laugh more. One of her first books (and one that I would highly recommend) is titled *"Stick a Geranium in Your Hat and Be Happy!"* (Johnson ,1987)[7]

I would recommend laughing more, as it is almost guaranteed to improve your mood, and at the same time strengthen the immune system. It has no negative side effects, and is available to us all, for free, all the time.

VII.   Healing Music

Music can be used as a therapy. It can assist to make your mind clearer, relieve anxiety and enhance your mood.

Music is created using different frequencies. These frequencies or wavelengths of sound have certain effects on the brain, emotions and ones resultant mood. For example, when someone listens to soothing music, they will feel more relaxed than when they are listening to loud, wild music. Loud and wild music can make the body more alert and even agitated.

To explain the different frequencies and their effect is rather complicated. You can read more in the following detailed study: *Auditory Beat Stimulation and its Effects on Cognition and Mood States*. (Chaieb, Wilpert, Reber & Fell, 2015)[8]

Music therapy has been used for centuries. Its effectiveness is described to us in 1 Samuel 16:14

–23, in the Bible. In this passage king Saul's mind was tormented at times but as soon as David would play on his harp for the king, Saul would feel better and the torment would subside. (NIV Bible, 1987)

Today music therapy is becoming popular to treat many health conditions.

According to an article by Beverly Merz (2015)[9] a growing body of research attests to the fact that music therapy can improve medical outcomes and quality of life in a variety of ways. Below are examples of these benefits:

- **Improves invasive procedures**: In controlled clinical trials of people having colonoscopies, cardiac angiography, and knee surgery, those who listened to music before their procedure had reduced anxiety and a reduced need for sedatives. Those who listened to music in the operating room reported less discomfort during their procedure. Hearing music in the recovery room lowered the use of opioid painkillers.
- **Reduces side effects of cancer therapy**: Listening to music reduces anxiety associated with chemotherapy and radiotherapy. It can also quell nausea and vomiting for patients receiving chemotherapy.
- **Aids pain relief:** Music therapy has been tested in patients ranging from those with intense acute pain to those with chronic pain from arthritis. Overall, music therapy

decreases pain perception, reduces the amount of pain medication needed, helps relieve depression, and gives people a sense of better control over their pain.

I often listen to music produced with healing in mind, to alleviate stress, anxiety and even tiredness.

There are two particular artists that I really enjoyed as mentioned already. The first was Jonathan Goldman and his *Holy Harmony* album. The second was Michael Tyrrell of Wholetones and his *Healing Frequencies Music Project*. Both have written about their music and how they developed the sounds and frequencies specifically for healing purposes

Listening to music could help to create an environment that is conducive to health and improve your overall well-being.

15. Conclusion

When I started my journey, I didn't anticipate the range of issues that would unfold along the way, issues that would lead to my healing both physically and emotionally. At the time, an alternative to chemotherapy and radiation was not considered a wise choice and was completely unsupported by the medical industry and general public consensus.

I had to search hard to gain an understanding of what it would take to restore health in my body. I am very grateful for those who have pioneered the way, and whose works I could discover and assemble into a comprehensive and coherent path.

I have tried my best to share my path in this book, which hopefully has left anyone afflicted by this disease with hope that it can be overcome, This hope arising from a series of protocols and methods that have been proven by myself and others as viable and workable.

The aim of my healing journey was not only to lengthen my life but also to have a good quality of life, even while I was in the process of healing. I believe I have achieved this, and I hope this was conveyed adequately.

We are all on a journey here on earth. From the day that we open our eyes, we start to experience life and learn new skills. We are deeply impacted by our early experiences and nutrition, which can impact our health positively or negatively. Later on we concentrate on gaining skills to survive financially, and often neglect the skills required for a healthy social and emotional life.

It is up to us to open our minds to new ideas and new ways. I have learned much during my journey out of cancer, and through this I have developed a passions to continue learning and gaining greater understanding about what is best to sustain the health of myself, my family and others, in the long term. This extends to nutrition, the emotions, natural anti-cancer treatments and the spirit.

I believe that no circumstance, difficulty or sickness is ever a waste of time and that everything that happens to us can work out for the best. Each one decides how difficulties will shape their lives for the future. We can allow them to propel us forward through what we learn from them, or we can remain stagnant.

In my case, I was in a situation that can and often leads to suffering and death. Those trained in the war on cancer, the oncologists, were of the view I would die within five years if I did not follow the conventional medical path. However, this was not to be, and through all the healing modalities I followed, I wasn't only healed physically but also became a better mother and person.

Along the way I decided to value and cherish every moment of life. I received a tremendous amount of emotional healing and stopped believing the lies that held me back from experiencing life with a sense of equanimity and strength. Through this, I enjoyed seeing my son grow into a beautiful young man, and all the way I was able to care for him and be fully involved in his upbringing.

I gained knowledge to advance my health through a holistic approach of concentrating on body, soul, spirit and mind. I can truly say that I have more energy now at sixty-one than I had in my mid-forties. My skin has changed from being red, dry, flaky and itchy - to natural. It is easy for me to live in my own skin now. My mind feels sound and at peace.

Having believed that it was time to share my journey with others, I wrote as comprehensively as possible about my experience. People need to know that there are alternatives for healing cancer. The diagnosis of cancer is on the increase, even among younger people (many in their forties). The option most frequently offered to them is still the conventional treatment of chemotherapy and radiation.

I would like to conclude with some verses from Psalm 103:1-5 (Amplified Bible, 2015). I read this passage often and it became one of my favourite scriptures because it reveals to me God's wonderful love and mercy for us.

Bless and affectionately praise the Lord, O my soul,

And all that is (deep) within me, bless His holy name.

Bless and affectionately praise the Lord, O my soul,
And do not forget any of His benefits;

Who forgives all your sins, Who heals all your diseases;

Who redeems your life from the pit, Who crowns you (lavishly) with loving kindness and tender mercy;

Who satisfies your years with good things,So that your youth is renewed like the (soaring) eagle.

Acknowledgements.

I could not have written this book without the wonderful support and assistance of my husband, Bruce. He believes, along with me, that this is a message that needs to get out into the world. Not only did he allow me the time to write, but he faithfully edited every piece that I wrote. He was also a tremendous help with the monumental task of getting the referencing correct.

I want to dedicate special thanks to my friend Suret Morkel, whom I got to know through her practice at Innerfruits. I was introduced to high-dose vitamin C drips and the benefits of them at this practice. Suret also supplied me with the ingredients necessary for the high-dose intravenous vitamin C drips, so I could use them at a nursing clinic, conveniently located near my home.

Much gratitude goes to my friend Pat, who counselled me, advised me, and faithfully prayed with me. I am so privileged to know Pat, a women with so much godly wisdom.

I am thankful for Joy, who started the Healing Rooms here in Melkbosstrand after she was diagnosed with breast cancer and decided against the conventional treatment. I appreciate the prayers that were prayed on my behalf, by all the prayer warriors. I met Sara Bock at this venue, who became a very good friend. I am so grateful for her joy, love and enthusiasm. To this day we still meet and pray, dance and sing together. This was, and still is, an important part of my healing.

Thanks to Dr Herman Spies, integrative medical doctor, who gave me the initial guidelines and procedures to natural healing and helped instil the hope of achieving this. He practises, and helps many, despite the scepticism from the conventional medical fraternity.

I am forever grateful for the nursing clinic that was opened, here in Melkbosstrand, just at the time that I needed to do the vitamin C drips. Sister St Claire was always so gentle and compassionate, and managed to insert the drips successfully without hurting me.

I am so grateful for my son, who was my inspiration to live. He encouraged me often by saying, "Mom, you must write it down," when I would share some healing revelation with him. He is truly living up to his name, Jonathan - gift from God. He continues to provide Bruce and I with lots of joy, as he grows in stature and wisdom.

A special thanks to Colleen, who has been a friend for 35 years. She is such a good listener and, after absorbing the issue for a while, would always come up with very wise advice. She started my emotional journey by lending me a book called *The Journey*, by Brandon Bays, which covers the importance of healing the emotions to heal cancer. She also gave me *The China Study*, by Colin Campbell, to listen to. This encouraged me to initially go on a completely vegan diet. Only much later did I discover the full benefit of a vegan diet for at least the first six months of any cancer treatment.

I thank my wonderful mother, who overcame ovarian cancer 15 years ago. She gave my decision to go the alternative healing route 100 per cent support. She is truly an example to me in so many areas of life, especially her unconditional love, determination and the strength of her faith in God.

Another friend I need to thank is Elizabeth, who was very involved with the birth of this book. She has encouraged me strongly to write with more feeling, and to draw my readers in to feel what I felt and experienced.

I also thank many other friends and family who supported me and prayed for me during this time. I thank my mom-in-law, Marie, for her kindness and love, and who faithfully put my name on the prayer list at her church.

Almost last, but not least, I have to thank Carri Kuhn, my editor, who patiently worked through my writings and assisted me greatly in making this book more professional.

Lastly, but most importantly, I want to thank my Creator and Heavenly Father, who led me on this journey and ultimately made the healing possible. God brought about physical healing but also spiritual and emotional healing. He provided every single thing that I needed on this journey. So the verse below has become true in my life.

"And we know that in all things God works for the good of those who love him, who have been called according to his purpose." (Romans 8:28, NIV Study Bible, 1985)

Addendum A.
Parasite Cleanse Handy Chart
Chart by Dr Hulda Clarck (2018)[4]

The 18 day program is as follows:

Day	Black Walnut Hull Tincture Strength Dose	WormwoodCapsule (200-300mg)	Clove Capsule 500mg
	1 time per day, like before a meal, in 1/2 cup of water	capsules 1 time per day, on empty stomach (before meal)	capsules 3 times a per day, like at mealtime
1	1 drop (or 1 capsule)	1	1,1,1
2	2 drops (or 1 capsule)	1	2,2,2
3	3 drops (or 1 capsule)	2	3,3,3
4	4 drops (or 1 capsule)	2	3,3,3

5	5 drops (or 1 capsule)	3	3,3,3
6	2 tsp. (or 2 capsules)	3	3,3,3
7	Now once a week	4	3,3,3
8		4	3,3,3
9		5	3,3,3
10		5	3,3,3
11		6	3
12		6	Now once a week
13	2 tsp. (or 2 capsules)	7	
14		7	
15		7	
16		7	
17		Now once a week	
18			3

After day 18 you do not need to keep a strict schedule, but instead may choose any day of the week to take all the parasite program ingredients.

Continue on the Maintenance Parasite Program, indefinitely, to prevent re-infection.

For a maintenance programme take once a week:

- 2 tsp black walnut tincture
- 7 wormwood capsules
- 3 cloves

References

Chapter 2:
1. Mayoclinic.org. (1998). Mammogram - Mayo Clinic. [online] Available at: https://www.mayoclinic.org/tests-procedures/mammogram/about/pac-20384806 [Accessed 3 Jun. 2018].

Chapter 3:
1. UCSF Medical Center.(2002). Breast Cancer Risk Factors. [online] Available at: https://www.ucsfhealth.org/education/breast_ cancer_risk_factors [Accessed 3 Jun. 2018].
2. Harris HR, Willett WC, Vaidya RL, Michels KB. (2017, March 1). An adolescent and early adulthood dietary pattern associated with inflammation and the incidence of breast cancer. Cancer research. 2017;77(5):1179-1187.doi:10. 1158/0008-5472.CAN-16-2273. (Discussion, para. 7) Available at: https://www.ncbi.nlm.nih.gov/pmc/articles/ PMC5335878/ [Accessed 3 Jun. 2018].
3. Huang, X. (PhD). (2008, August 9). Does iron have a role in breast cancer?. The Lancet Oncology, 9(8), pp.803-807. (Conclusion, para. 1) Available at https://www.ncbi.nlm.nih.gov/pmc/articles/PMC2577284/ [Accessed 3 Jun. 2018].
4. Brownstein, D. (M.D). (2014) Iodine: Why You Need It, Why You Can't Live Without It. Colorado: Selene River Press.
5. Rupp, J. (2004). Bilharzia. [online] Escargot.ch. Available at: http://www.escargot.ch/personel/schisto.htm [Accessed 3 Jun. 2018].
6. Spies, H. (M.B.Ch.B). (2018). Biopuncture, Sports Injuries, Chronic Pain - Treatments - Holistic Treatments in Cape Town, Alternative Health Treatments, Holistic Medicine Treatments in Cape Town - The Quantec Scan. [online] Drspies.com. (para. 1-2). Available at: http://www.drspies.com/treatments_details.php?id=12 [Accessed 3 Jun. 2018].
7. Jimenez, T. (M.D). (2015, November 16). [The Truth About Cancer]. Detoxification for Cancer Patients - Dr. Tony Jimenez, MD || A Global Quest Video Clips. [online] YouTube. Available at: https://www.youtube.com/watch?v=GBpN1Q07nS8 [Accessed 3 Jun. 2018].
8. Heid, M. (2014, December). How stress affects cancer risk. [online] MD Anderson Cancer Center. (Not all stress is equally

harmful, para. 1-3).Available at: https://www.mdanderson.org/publications/focused-on-health/ december-2014/how-stress-affects-cancer-risk.html.html [Accessed 3 Jun. 2018].

Chapter 4:
1. Pasquini, M. and Biondi, M. (2007). Clinical Practice and Epidemiology in Mental Health, 3(1), p.2. "Depression in cancer patients: a critical review" (Background section. Line no's 5-7) US. National Library of Medicine. Available at https://www.ncbi.nlm.nih.gov/pmc/articles/PMC1797173/ [Accessed 3 Jun. 2018].
2. Morgan, G, Ward, R & Barton, M. (2004). "The contribution of cytotoxic chemotherapy to 5-year survival in adult malignancies". Clin Oncol (R Coll Radiol)2004;16:549-60
3. Gawler, I (Dr) OAM, BVSc, MCouns&HS. (2007). Prepared with assistance from Dr Craig Hassed MBBS, FRACGP, Senior Lecturer, Department of General Practice, Monash University.(June 2007). "Cancer, lifestyle and chemotherapy" [online] Iangawler.com. (par. Chemotherapy and breast cancer - a specific example. Page 10.) Available at: https://iangawler.com/info/ articles/Cancer%20lifestyle%20and%20chemotherapy.pdf?x46763 [Accessed 3 Jun. 2018].
4. Segelov, E. (2006, Feb). The emperor's new clothes - can chemotherapy survive?. Australian Prescriber, 29(1), pp.2-3. (Para 7) Available at http://www.nps.org.au/australian - prescriber/ articles/the-emperor-s-new-clothes-can-chemotherapy-survive [Accessed 3 Jun. 2018].
5. Duric, VM., Stockler, MR., Heritier, S., Boyle, F., Beith, J., Sullivan, A., Wilcken, N., Coates, AS., Simes, RJ., (2005, Nov). Annals of Oncology. U.S. National Library of Medicine. "Patients' preferences for adjuvant chemotherapy in early breast cancer: what makes AC and CMF worthwhile now?". (Para 3) Available at https://www.ncbi.nlm.nih.gov/pubmed/ 16126738 [Accessed 3 Jun. 2018].
6. CancerCenter.com. (2017). Breast Cancer Survival Statistics | CTCA. [online] Available at: https://www.cancercenter.com/breast-cancer/statistics/tab/breast-cancer-survival-statistics [Accessed 3 Jun. 2018].
7. Cancer.org. (2017). Chemotherapy for Breast Cancer. [online] Available at: https://www.cancer.org/cancer/breast-

cancer/treatment/chemotherapy-for-breast-cancer.html [Accessed 3 Jun. 2018].
8. Irwin, K. (2012). Radiation generates cancer stem cells from less aggressive breast cancer cells. [online] UCLA Newsroom. Available at: http://newsroom.ucla.edu/releases/ radiation-treatments-generate-229002 [Accessed 3 Jun. 2018].
9. John Hopkins Medicine. Report on study by Greg Semenza MD et al. Hopkinsmedicine.org. (2017, February). Scientists Identify Chain Reaction That Shields Breast Cancer Stem Cells From Chemotherapy - 02/22/2017. [online] Available at: https://www.hopkinsmedicine.org/news/media/releases/scientists_identify_chain_reaction_that_shields_breast_cancer_stem_cells_from_chemotherapy [Accessed 3 Jun. 2018].

Chapter 5:
1. Ohno, S., Ohno, Y., Suzuki, N., Soma, G. and Inoue, M. (2008). High-dose Vitamin C (Ascorbic Acid) Therapy in the Treatment of Patients with Advanced Cancer. (Historical Background on high dose vitamin C. Para 1) [online] Ar.iiarjournals.org. Available at: http://ar.iiarjournals.org/content/29/3/809.full [Accessed 3 Jun. 2018].
2. Creagan, ET. and Et.al (1979). Failure of High-Dose Vitamin C (Ascorbic Acid) Therapy to Benefit Patients with Advanced Cancer — A Controlled Trial | NEJM. [online] New England Journal of Medicine. Available at: https:// www.nejm.org/doi/full/10.1056/ NEJM197909273011303 [Accessed 3 Jun. 2018].
3. Chen' Q., Espey, MG., Krishna, MC., Mitchell, JB., Corpe, CP. , Buettner, GR., Shacter, E., Levine, M.: (2005) "Pharmacologic ascorbic acid concentrations selectively kill cancer cells: action as a pro-drug to deliver hydrogen peroxide to tissues". Proc Natl Acad Sci USA 102: 13604-13609.
4. Chen Q, Espey MG, Sun AY, Lee JH, Krishna MC, Shacter E, Choyke PL, Pooput C,Kirk KL, Buettner GR, Levine M (2007) "Ascorbate in pharmacologic concentrations selectively generates ascorbate radical and hydrogen peroxide in extracellular fluid in vivo". Proc Natl Acad Sci USA 104: 8749-8754
5. Pauling, LC. (Dr.) (1986)., How to Live Longer and Feel Better
6. Riordan, NH., Riordan, HD., Meng, X., Li, Y. and Jackson, JA. (1995). Intravenous ascorbate as a tumor cytotoxic

chemotherapeutic agent. - PubMed - NCBI. [online] Ncbi.nlm.nih.gov. Available at: https://www.ncbi.nlm.nih.gov/pubmed/7609676 [Accessed 3 Jun. 2018].
7. Doctoryourself.com.Riordan Clinic Research Institute (2013, February)"The Riordan IVC Protocol for Adjunctive Cancer Care Intravenous Ascorbate as a Chemotherapeutic and Biological Response Modifying Agent" (Page 2) [online] Available at: http://www.doctoryourself.com/RiordanIVC.pdf [Accessed 3 Jun. 2018].
8. Huber, C. (2014). Breast Cancer Patients' Treatment Choices and Outcomes in a Naturopathic Clinic. [online] Opastonline.com. Available at: http://www.opastonline.com/wp-content/uploads/2017/02/Breast-Cancer-Patients-Treatment-Choices-and-Outcomes-in-a-Naturopathic-Clinic-ijcrt-17-007.pdf [Accessed 3 Jun. 2018].

Chapter 6
1. Ravindran, J., Prasad, S. & Aggarwal, B.B. AAPS J (2009) 11: 495. https://doi.org/10.1208/s12248-009-9128-x [Accessed 3 Jun. 2018].
2. Adamo, C. (2017). The Ionic Foot Detox: Fact or Myth?. [online] Pacific College of Oriental Medicine. Available at: https://www.pacificcollege.edu/news/blog/2015/04/24/ionic-foot-detox-fact-or-myth [Accessed 3 Jun. 2018].
3. Your Rife Machine History Educational Website. Rifevideos.com. (n.d.). Dr. Rife's Newspaper Articles. [online] Available at: http://rifevideos.com/doctors_who_used_the_rife_machine_on_their_patients.html [Accessed 3 Jun. 2018].

Chapter 7:
1. Christopoulos, F., Msaouel, P. and Koutsilieris, M. (2015). The role of the insulin-like growth factor-1 system in breast cancer. Molecular Cancer, 14(1), p.43. Available at https://molecular-cancer.biomedcentral.com/articles/ 10.1186/s12943-015-0291-7[Accessed 3 Jun. 2018].
2. Insulin-like growth factor 1 (IGF1), IGF binding protein 3 (IGFBP3), and breast cancer risk: pooled individual data analysis of 17 prospective studies. (2010). The Lancet Oncology, 11(6), pp.530-542. Available at https://www.ncbi.nlm.nih.gov/pubmed/20472501[Accessed 3 Jun. 2018].
3. Rigby, B. (n.d.). Does Meat Cause Cancer? Revisiting the Meat, IGF-1, and Cancer Connection | Sara Gottfried MD. [online] Saragottfriedmd.com. Available at: http://www.

saragottfriedmd.com/does-meat-cause-cancer-revisiting-the-meat-igf-1-and-cancer-connection [Accessed 3 Jun. 2018].
4. Cellarier, E., Durando, X., Vasson, MP., Farges, MC., Demiden, A., Maurizis, JC., Madelmont, JC., Chollet, P., Cellarier, E, e. (2003). Methionine dependency and cancer treatment. - PubMed - NCBI. [online] Ncbi.nlm.nih.gov. Available at: https://www.ncbi.nlm.nih.gov/pubmed/ 14585259 [Accessed 3 Jun. 2018].
5. Greger, M. (FACLM,MD). (2013). Starving Cancer with Methionine Restriction | NutritionFacts.org. [online] Nutritionfacts.org. Available at: https://nutritionfacts.org/video/starving-cancer-with-methionine-restriction [Accessed 10 Jun. 2018].
6. Lamb, R., Harrison, H., Smith, D., Townsend, P., Jackson, T., Ozsvari, B., Martinez-Outschoorn, U., Pestell, R., Howell, A., Lisanti, M. and Sotgia, F. (2015). Targeting tumor-initiating cells: Eliminating anabolic cancer stem cells with inhibitors of protein synthesis or by mimicking caloric restriction. [online] Oncotarget. 2015;6(7):4585-4601. Available at: http://www.oncotarget.com/index.php? journal=oncotarget&page=article&op=view&path[]= 3278&path[]= 6346 [Accessed 1 Jun. 2018].
7. Whitbread, D. (MScN). (2018). Top 10 Foods Highest in Methionine. [online] myfooddata. Available at: https://www.myfooddata.com/articles/high-methionine-foods.php [Accessed 1 Jun. 2018].
8. Gear, J., Brodribb, A., Ware, A. and Mannt, J. (1981). Fibre and bowel transit times. British Journal of Nutrition, [online] 45(01), p.77. Available at: https://www.cambridge.org/core/journals/ british-journal-of-nutrition/article/fibre-and-bowel-transit-times/ BF3233807EE354316C209086EFC88869. [Accessed 3 Jun. 2018].
9. Wlassoff, W. (Dr). (2015, July). From Mouth To Bowel Movement: What Your Food Transit Time Says About Your Health | Gastrointestinal Disorders articles | Body & Health Conditions center | SteadyHealth.com. [online] Steadyhealth.com. Available at: https://www.steadyhealth.com/articles/from-mouth-to-bowel-movement-what-your-food-transit-time-says-about-your-health?show_all=1 [Accessed 1 Jun. 2018].
10. Nutrition Insight. (2016). Transit time of Food is Key to Digestive Health, Claims New Study. [online] Available at: http://www.nutritioninsight.com/news/Transit-time-of-Food-is-

Key-to-Digestive-Health-Claims-New-Study.html [Accessed 1 Jun. 2018].
11. National Cancer Institute. (2012). Cruciferous Vegetables and Cancer Prevention. [online] Available at: https://www.cancer.gov/about-cancer/causes-prevention/risk/diet/cruciferous-vegetables-fact-sheet [Accessed 1 Jun. 2018].
12. Anand, P., Kunnumakkara, A., Sundaram, C., Harikumar, K., Tharakan, S., Lai, O., Sung, B. and Aggarwal, B. (2008). Cancer is a Preventable Disease that Requires Major Lifestyle Changes. Pharmaceutical Research, [online] 25(9), pp.2200-2200. Available at: https://www.ncbi.nlm.nih.gov/pubmed/18626751 [Accessed 1 Jun. 2018].
13. Watson, G., Beaver, L., Williams, D., Dashwood, R. and Ho, E. (2013). Phytochemicals from Cruciferous Vegetables, Epigenetics, and Prostate Cancer Prevention. The AAPS Journal, [online] 15(4), pp.951-961. Available at: https://www.ncbi.nlm.nih.gov/pmc/articles/PMC3787240/. [Accessed 3 Jun. 2018].
14. Weng, J., Tsai, C., Kulp, S. and Chen, C. (2008). Indole-3-carbinol as a chemopreventive and anti-cancer agent. Cancer Letters, [online] 262(2), pp.153-163. Available at: https://www.ncbi.nlm.nih.gov/pmc/articles/PMC2814317/.[Accessed 3 Jun. 2018].
15. Royston, K. and Tollefsbol, T. (2015). The Epigenetic Impact of Cruciferous Vegetables on Cancer Prevention. Current Pharmacology Reports, 1(1), pp.46-51. Available at: https://link.springer.com/article/10.1007/s40495-014-0003-9. [Accessed 3 Jun. 2018].
16. Talalay, P. and Fahey, J. (2001). Phytochemicals from Cruciferous Plants Protect against Cancer by Modulating Carcinogen Metabolism. The Journal of Nutrition, [online] 131(11), pp.3027S-3033S. Available at: https://academic.oup.com/jn/article/131/11/3027S/4686710. [Accessed 3 Jun. 2018].
17. Healthbeckon.com. (2014). 20 Best Fiber Rich Vegetables You Should Include In Your Diet. [online] Available at: https://www.healthbeckon.com/fiber-rich-vegetables/ [Accessed 10 Jun. 2018].
18. Whfoods.com. (2018). Eating Healthy with Cruciferous Vegetables. [online] Available at: http://www.whfoods.com/genpage.php?tname=btnews&dbid=126 [Accessed 10 Jun. 2018].

19. Greger, M. (MD. FACLM). (2016). How to Cook Broccoli | NutritionFacts.org. [online] NutritionFacts.org. Available at: https://nutritionfacts.org/2016/02/09/how-to-cook-broccoli/ [Accessed 10 Jun. 2018].
20. Kristo, A., Klimis-Zacas, D. and Sikalidis, A. (2016). Protective Role of Dietary Berries in Cancer. Antioxidants, [online] 5(4), p.37. Available at: http://www.mdpi.com/2076-3921/5/4/37. [Accessed 3 Jun. 2018].
21. Project Principal is Yanyun Zhoa, O. (n.d.). Fact Sheets for blackberries, blueberries, raspberries, and strawberries ~ Connecting Berry Health Benefit Researchers. [online] Berryhealth.fst.oregonstate.edu. Available at: http://berryhealth.fst.oregonstate.edu/health_healing/fact_she ets [Accessed 10 Jun. 2018].
22. Russell, L., Mazzio, E., Badisa, R., Zhu, Z., Agharahimi, M., Oriaku, E. and Goodman, C. (2012). Autoxidation of Gallic Acid Induces ROS-dependent Death in Human Prostate Cancer LNCaP Cells. [online] Ar.iiarjournals.org. Available at: http://ar.iiarjournals.org/content/32/5/1595.long [Accessed 10 Jun. 2018].
23. Hammer, D. (2009). The ORAC Rating Table!. [online] Aging-no-more.com. Available at: http://www.aging-no-more.com/orac-rating.html [Accessed 10 Jun. 2018].
24. Environmental Working Group (2017). The 2017 Dirty Dozen: Strawberries, Spinach Top EWG's List of Pesticides in Produce. [online] Available at: https://www.ewg.org/release/2017-dirty-dozen-strawberries-spinach-top-ewgs-list-pesticides-produce#.Wx0o-LixWUn [Accessed 10 Jun. 2018].
25. Fassa, P. (2009). Apricot Seeds Kill Cancer Cells without Side Effects. [online] NaturalNews. Available at: https://www.naturalnews.com/027088_cancer_laetrile_cure.html [Accessed 10 Jun. 2018].
26. Gerson Institute. (2011). The Gerson Therapy | Gerson Institute. [online] Available at: https://gerson.org/gerpress/the-gerson-therapy/ [Accessed 10 Jun. 2018].
27. Mercola (Dr) (2003). Better than Wheatgrass: Raw Veggie Juice and Sprouts. [online] Waking Times. Available at: http://www.wakingtimes.com/2013/05/30/better-than-wheatgrass-raw-veggie-juice-and-sprouts [Accessed 10 Jun. 2018]. [Accessed 3 Jun. 2018].
28. Brown S.E. (DR), (2015). 10 Steps to Stronger Digestion. [online] Better Bones. Available at: https://www.betterbones.com/bone-nutrition/better-digestion/ [Accessed 10 Jun. 2018].

29. Oasis Integrative Medicine. (2015). The Dirty Dozen™ – 12 Foods You Should Avoid Eating. [online] Available at: http://www.oasismedicine.com/blog-posts/dirty-dozen-12-foods-avoid-eating/ [Accessed 10 Jun. 2018].
30. Bell, R.S. (Dr). (n.d.). Video - Why You Must Eliminate Pesticides in Food When Treating Cancer. [online] The Truth About Cancer. Available at: https://dev.thetruthaboutcancer.com/video-pesticides-in-food-treating-cancer/ [Accessed 10 Jun. 2018].
31. Tasty Yummies. (n.d.). 10 Benefits to Drinking Warm Lemon Water Every Morning - Tasty Yummies. [online] Available at: http://tasty-yummies.com/10-benefits-to-drinking-warm-lemon-water-every-morning/ [Accessed 10 Jun. 2018].
32. Mercola.com. (n.d.). Intermittent Fasting Infographic. [online] Available at: https://www.mercola.com/infographics/intermittent-fasting.htm [Accessed 10 Jun. 2018].
33. McGruther, J. (n.d.). What Veg*ns Can Learn from Traditional Foods. [online] Nourished Kitchen. (1. To soak, sour or sprout grains, legumes, nuts, seeds and beans.) Available at: https://nourishedkitchen.com/what-vegns-can-learn-from-traditional-foods [Accessed 10 Jun. 2018].
34. The Weston A. Price Foundation. (n.d.). Soy Alert!. [online] Available at: https://www.westonaprice.org/soy-alert [Accessed 10 Jun. 2018].
35. Organixx. (n.d.). Bone Broth Protein Powder | Organixx. [online] Available at: https://organixx.com/bone-broth-protein [Accessed 10 Jun. 2018].
36. Rawblend.com.au. (n.d.). Green Smoothies - Why They're So Good For You - Raw Blend. [online] Available at: https://www.rawblend.com.au/green-smoothies.html [Accessed 10 Jun. 2018].
37. Dr. Axe. (n.d.). 7 Health Benefits of Grass-Fed Butter Nutrition - Dr. Axe. [online] Available at: https://draxe.com/ grass-fed-butter-nutrition [Accessed 10 Jun. 2018].
38. Dr. Axe. (n.d.). Coconut Oil Benefits + How to Get the Benefits of Coconut Oil - Dr. Axe. [online] Available at: https://draxe.com/coconut-oil-benefits [Accessed 10 Jun. 2018].
39. Ravindran, J., Prasad, S. and Aggarwal, B. (2009). Curcumin and Cancer Cells: How Many Ways Can Curry Kill Tumor Cells Selectively?. The AAPS Journal, [online] 11(3), pp.495-510. Available at: https://link.springer.

com/article/10.1208%2Fs12248-009-9128-x. [Accessed 3 Jun. 2018].
40. Jockers, D. (DC, MS, CSCS). (n.d.). Are You Eating These 8 Nutrients That Block Cancer Metastasis?. [online] The Truth About Cancer. Available at: https://thetruthabout cancer.com/nutrients-block-cancer-metastasis [Accessed 10 Jun. 2018].

Chapter 8
1. Hopegood, R. (2015). What does your gut do and how can you keep your digestive system healthy?. [online] Mirror. Available at: https://www.mirror.co.uk/lifestyle/health/what-your-gut-how-can-6164204 [Accessed 10 Jun. 2018].
2. Carpenter, S. (Dr). (2012). That gut feeling. Monitor on Psychology, [online] (Vol. 43 no. 8), p.50. Available at: http://www.apa.org/monitor/2012/09/gut-feeling.aspx [Accessed 10 Jun. 2018].
3. Wardill, HR. and Gibson, RJ. (2017). How our gut bacteria affect cancer risk and response to treatment. [online] The Conversation. Available at: https://theconversation. com/how-our-gut-bacteria-affect-cancer-risk-and-response-to-treatment-75699 [Accessed 10 Jun. 2018].
4. Brubaker, J. (2017). The Breast Microbiome: A Role for Probiotics in Breast Cancer Prevention. [online] Asm.org. Available at: http://www.asm.org/index.php/general-science-blog/item/6663-the-breast-microbiome-a-role-for-probiotics-in-breast-cancer-prevention [Accessed 10 Jun. 2018].
5. Mercola, J., (Dr). (2012). How Your Gut Flora Influences Your Health. [online] Mercola.com. Available at: http:// articles.mercola.com/sites/articles/archive/2012/06/27/probiotics-gut-health-impact.aspx [Accessed 10 Jun. 2018].
6. Mercola, J., (Dr). (2016). Gut Microbiome Influences Your Mental and Physical Health. [online] Mercola.com. Available at: https://articles.mercola.com/sites/articles/archive/2016/01/07/how-gut-microbiome-influences-health.aspx [Accessed 10 Jun. 2018].

Chapter 9
1. The American Cancer Society medical and editorial content team (2016). Parasites that can lead to cancer | American Cancer Society. [online] Cancer.org. Available at: https:// www.cancer.org/cancer/cancer-causes/infectious-agents/

infections-that-can-lead-to-cancer/parasites.html [Accessed 10 Jun. 2018].
2. Rupp, J. (2004). Environmental management: Bilharzia. [online] Escargot.ch. Available at: http://www.escargot.ch/personel/schisto.htm [Accessed 10 Jun. 2018].
3. Meyers, A. (2013). 10 Signs You May Have A Parasite. [online] mindbodygreen. Available at: https://www.mindbodygreen.com/0-11321/10-signs-you-may-have-a-parasite.html [Accessed 10 Jun. 2018].
4. Clark, H., (Dr). (2018.). Dr. Hulda Clark's Herbal Parasite Cleanse for Beginners. [online] Drclark.net. Available at: http://www.drclark.net/cleanses/beginners/herbal-parasite-cleanse/parasite-chart-for-adults [Accessed 10 Jun. 2018].

Chapter 10
1. Wilson, L., (Dr). (2018). COFFEE ENEMAS (Chapter 3. Effects Of Coffee Enemas). [online] Drlwilson.com. Available at: https://www.drlwilson.com/articles/COFFEE%20ENEMA.HTM#CH3 [Accessed 10 Jun. 2018].
2. Coffee enema. (2016). Available at: https://en.wikipedia.org/wiki/Coffee_enema [Accessed 10 Jun. 2018].
3. Gerson, C. (n.d.). Scientific Basis of Coffee Enemas. [online] www.gerson.org. Available at: https://gerson.org/pdfs/How_Coffee_Enemas_Work.pdf [Accessed 10 Jun. 2018].

Chapter 11
1. Quizlet. (n.d.). Lymphatic System Flashcards. [online] Available at: https://quizlet.com/29396130/lymphatic-system-flash-cards [Accessed 10 Jun. 2018].
2. Showers, A. (2014). Lymphatic and Immune System of the Human Body | Mind Body and Soul. [online] Msaprilshowers.com. Available at: http://msaprilshowers.com/body/lymphatic-and-immune-system-of-the-human-body [Accessed 10 Jun. 2018].
3. Protocol-ID | TrulyHeal. (2018). Retrieved from https://trulyheal.com/ozone/ozone-therapy-for-infectious-diseases-lyme-hiv-hepatitis-c/protocol-id/
4. Wibbels, H. (2010). Self Lymph Drainage Massage. [video] Available at: https://www.youtube.com/watch?v=QA-wi0d7-Ro&t=87s [Accessed 10 Jun. 2018].
5. Spies, H., (Dr). (2017). Biopuncture, Sports Injuries, Chronic Pain - Treatments - Holistic Treatments in Cape Town,

Alternative Health Treatments, Holistic Medicine Treatments in Cape Town. [online] Drspies.com. Available at: https://www.drspies.com/treatments_details.php?id=24 [Accessed 10 Jun. 2018].
6. Mama, K. (2018). How to Make & Use Castor Oil Packs | Wellness Mama. Available at https://wellnessmama.com/35671/castor-oil-packs[Accessed 3 Jun. 2018].
7. Genuis, S., Beesoon, S., Birkholz, D., & Lobo, R. (2011). Human Excretion of Bisphenol A: Blood, Urine, and Sweat (BUS) Study. Available at ttps://www.ncbi.nlm.nih.gov/pmc/articles/PMC3255175[Accessed 3 Jun. 2018].
8. Ozone Sauna Therapy. (2017). "Ozone Sauna Therapy Information, Ozone Sauna Articles, and Ozone Sauna Therapy Studies" Available at http://www.oxygenhealingtherapies.com/ozone_sauna_therapy.htm [Accessed 3 Jun. 2018].
9. People who exercise on work days are happier, suffer less stress and are more productive. (2008). Available at http://www.dailymail.co.uk/news/article-1095783/People-exercise-work-days-happier-suffer-stress-productive.html#ixzz5DcEGMmRj [Accessed 3 Jun. 2018].
10. Mayo Clinic Staff (2013) "Exercise: 7 great reasons why exercise matters. Available at https://www.mayoclinic.org/healthy-lifestyle/fitness/in-depth/exercise/art-20048389 [Accessed 3 Jun. 2018].

Chapter 12
1. Brownstein,D.,(MD). "Iodine: Why You Need It, Why You Can't Live Without It" Paperback book 4th Edition (2009)
2. Brownstein,D., (MD). "Iodine: Why You Need It, Why You Can't Live Without It" Paperback book 4th Edition (2009) Page 80.
3. Brownstein,d.,(MD). "Iodine: Why You Need It, Why You Can't Live Without It" Paperback book 4th Edition (2009) Page 24.
4. How does the thyroid gland work?. (2015). para.1 & 10 Available at https://www.ncbi.nlm.nih.gov/pubmedhealth/PMH0072572/ [Accessed 3 Jun. 2018].
5. Aceves, C., Anguiano, B., & Delgado, G. (2005). Is Iodine A Gatekeeper of the Integrity of the Mammary Gland? Journal Of Mammary Gland Biology And Neoplasia, 10(2), 189-196. doi: 10.1007/s10911-005-5401-5. Available at https://link.

springer.com/article/10. 1007%2Fs10911- 005-5401-5 [Accessed 3 Jun. 2018].
6. Jacobs,E,. Do You Have Low Iodine?: The Link Between Iodine Deficiency & Cancer. Available at https://thetruth aboutcancer.com/low-iodine-cancer/ [Accessed 3 Jun. 2018].
7. Michael B. Schachter, M.D. (2005, August) "Iodine: Its Role In Health and Disease. Some New Exciting Concepts "(Introduction para. 2, Factors that Aggravate Iodine Insufficiency section, para. 4) Available at http:// www. mbschachter.com/iodine.htm [Accessed 3 Jun. 2018].

Chapter 13
1. Leaf, C., (2013) "Switch On Your Brain" (Paperback)
2. Pert, C.B., (1997) "Molecules of Emotion, The Science Behind Mind-Body Medicine" (Available in various printed and electronic formats)
3. Hay, Louise L., (2004) "You can Heal your Life" (Available in various printed and electronic formats)
4. Loyd, A., & Johnson, B. (2004) The Healing Codes - Unlocking the Cellular Sequence of Life (P135)
5. Lipton,B., (2005) "The Biology of Belief, Unleashing the Power of Consciousness Matter and Miracles"..Published by Hay House
6. Cohen, H., (2017, March) "10 Ways to Think More Positively" Baseline of Health Foundation. Available at https://jonbarron.org/happiness-mental-health/10-ways-think-more-positively [Accessed 3 Jun. 2018].

Chapter 14
1. Prince, J (2007) Destined to Reign: The Secret to Effortless Success, Wholeness and Victorious Living. Harrison House. Paperback
2. Editorial Team - The Health Site (2015, March) "10 ways praying actually benefits your health!" Available at http:// www.thehealthsite.com/diseases-conditions/10-ways-praying-actually-benefits-your-health-p114/ [Accessed 3 Jun. 2018].
3. Fancourt, D., Williamson, A., Carvalho,I., Steptoe, A., Dow, R., Lewis, I., (2016) ecancermedicalscience website "Singing modulates mood, stress, cortisol, cytokine and neuropeptide activity in cancer patients and carers". Available at https://ecancer.org/journal/10/631-singing-modulates-mood-stress-cortisol-cytokine-and-neuropeptide-activity-in-cancer-patients-and-carers.php [Accessed 3 Jun. 2018].

4. Bellert, JL. (1989) "Humor. A therapeutic approach in oncology nursing"(US National Librabry of History, Abstract. Available at https://www.ncbi.nlm.nih.gov/pubmed/2713839 [Accessed 3 Jun. 2018].
5. Gorman, J. (Citing Dr. Dunbar,R. an evolutionary psychologist at Oxford) (2011, September), "Scientists Hint at Why Laughter Feels So Good" Available at https://www.nytimes.com/2011/09/14/science/14laughter.html [Accessed 3 Jun. 2018].
6. Markham, H. (2014, November) "You Asked: Does Laughing Have Real Health Benefits?" (para 5&6. Citing the work of Dr Berk, L.) Available at http://www.dr-lee-berk.com/blog.html [Accessed 3 Jun. 2018].
7. Johnson, B. (1987) "Stick a Geranium in Your Hat and Be Happy!" Paperback. Published by Thomas Nelson.
8. Chaieb, L., Wipert, E., Reber, T., and Fell, J. (2015, May) US National Library of Medicine. "Auditory Beat Stimulation and its Effects on Cognition and Mood States" Available at https://www.ncbi.nlm.nih.gov/pmc/articles/PMC4428073 [Accessed 3 Jun. 2018].
9. Merz, B. (Executive ED), Harvard Women's Health Watch (2015, November) Harvard Medical School "Healing through music" (The Evidence for Music Therapy para) Available at https://www.health.harvard.edu/ blog/healing-through-music-201511058556 [Accessed 3 Jun. 2018].

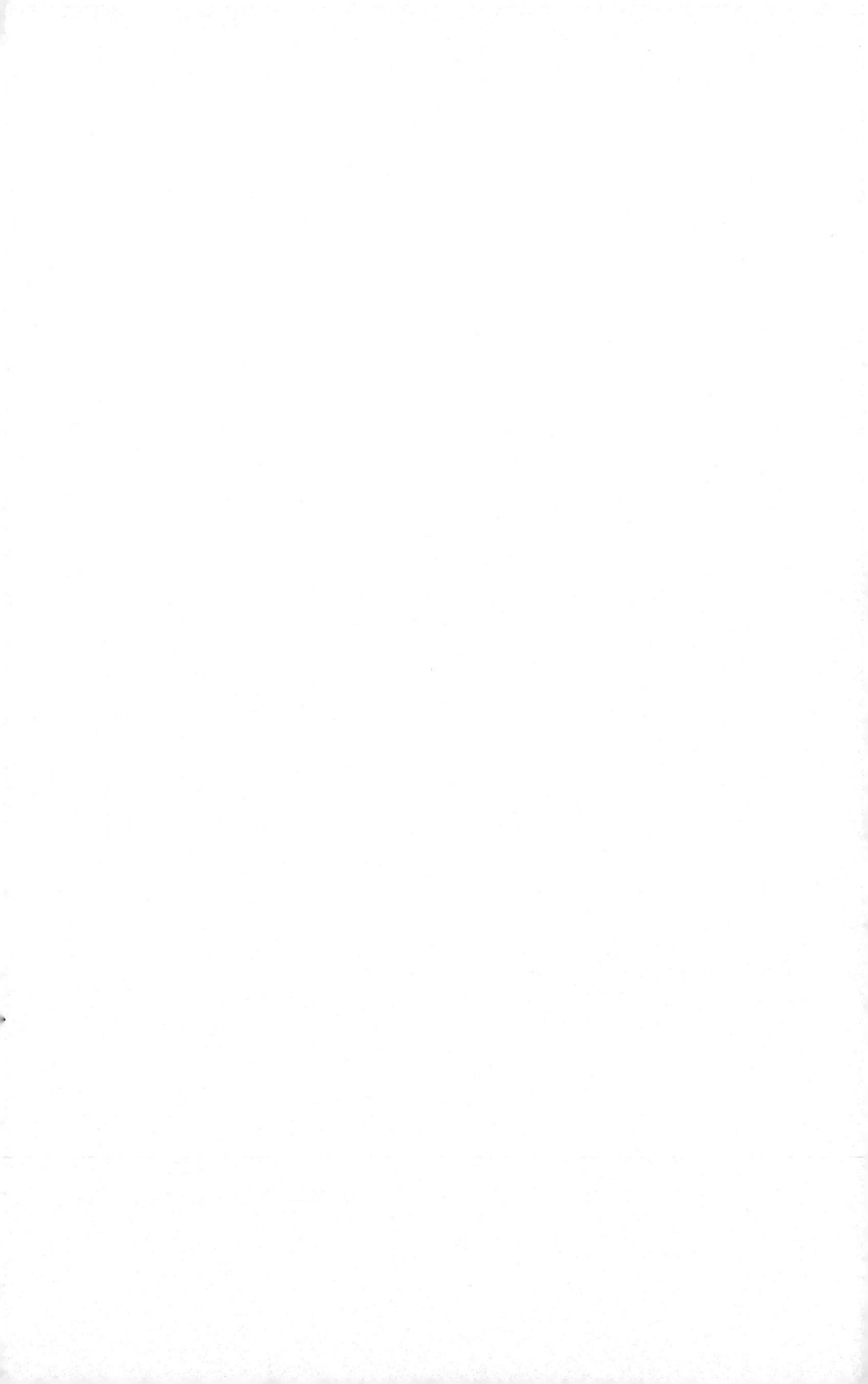

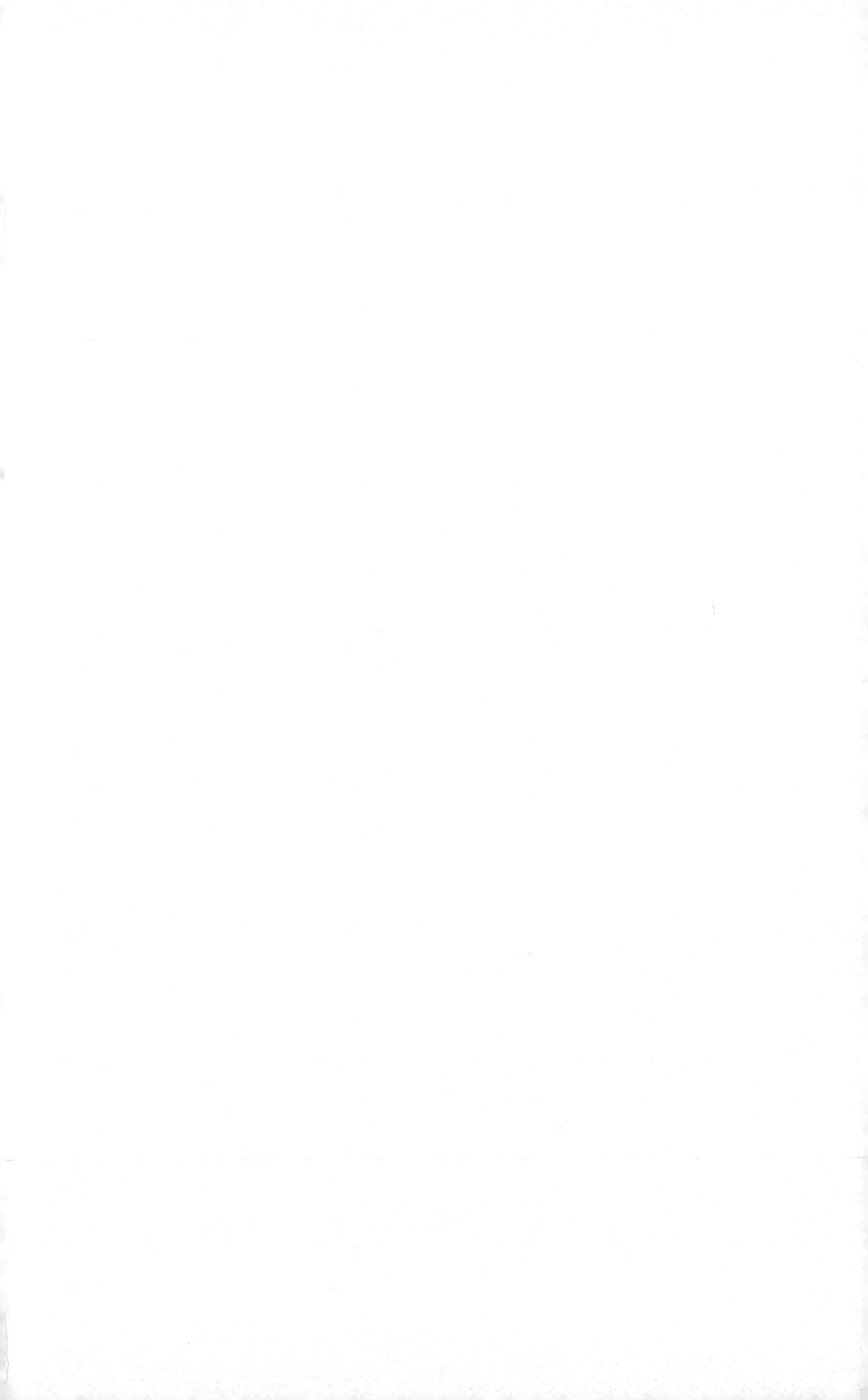

Printed in Great Britain
by Amazon